AF763523

Multi-Modality Neuroimaging Study on Neurobiological Mechanisms of Acupuncture

Jie Tian
Editor

Multi-Modality Neuroimaging Study on Neurobiological Mechanisms of Acupuncture

Springer

Editor
Jie Tian
CAS Key Laboratory of Molecular Imaging
Institute of Automation
Beijing
China

ISBN 978-981-10-4913-2 ISBN 978-981-10-4914-9 (eBook)
DOI 10.1007/978-981-10-4914-9

Library of Congress Control Number: 2017951645

© Springer Nature Singapore Pte Ltd. 2018
This work is subject to copyright. All rights are reserved by the Publisher, whether the whole or part of the material is concerned, specifically the rights of translation, reprinting, reuse of illustrations, recitation, broadcasting, reproduction on microfilms or in any other physical way, and transmission or information storage and retrieval, electronic adaptation, computer software, or by similar or dissimilar methodology now known or hereafter developed.
The use of general descriptive names, registered names, trademarks, service marks, etc. in this publication does not imply, even in the absence of a specific statement, that such names are exempt from the relevant protective laws and regulations and therefore free for general use.
The publisher, the authors and the editors are safe to assume that the advice and information in this book are believed to be true and accurate at the date of publication. Neither the publisher nor the authors or the editors give a warranty, express or implied, with respect to the material contained herein or for any errors or omissions that may have been made. The publisher remains neutral with regard to jurisdictional claims in published maps and institutional affiliations.

Printed on acid-free paper

This Springer imprint is published by Springer Nature
The registered company is Springer Nature Singapore Pte Ltd.
The registered company address is: 152 Beach Road, #21-01/04 Gateway East, Singapore 189721, Singapore

Contents

Early fMRI Studies of Acupuncture

1

Wei Qin, Lingmin Jin, and Jie Tian

1.1 Introduction

Acupuncture is the method of inserting needles into specific physiological acupoints with the purpose of addressing therapeutic requirements guided by the theory of traditional Chinese medicine (TCM). Acupuncture has been practiced clinically in China and Eastern Asia for more than 2000 years. According to the theory of TCM, the efficacy of acupuncture is attributed to deqi, which is a composite of unique sensations induced by acupuncture stimulation, and the functional specificity of given acupoints distributed throughout the body. In 1997, a National Institutes of Health consensus conference was held to assess the clinical use and effectiveness of acupuncture as a standalone or adjunct therapy for indications such as postoperative and chemotherapy-induced nausea, postoperative dental pain, and other conditions. This panel called for the conduct of additional high-quality randomized controlled trials of acupuncture (NIH Consensus Conference 1998). Since then, there has been an explosion of basic research studies and clinical applications of acupuncture around the world. Indeed, in 2014, the World Health Organization reported the use of acupuncture in a total of 183 countries (WHO 2014).

TCM purports that the therapeutic effects of acupuncture are mediated by the ability of acupoint stimulation to adjust an individual's qi and blood balance. However, this theory of balance regulation is not entirely compatible with contemporary biomedical information. Accordingly, the exact underlying biological mechanisms of acupuncture remain unclear. There is a need for research to integrate what is known regarding various acupoints into the practice and context of modern medicine. In 1998, Cho proposed a conceptual relationship between the brain, organs,

W. Qin • L. Jin
School of Life Sciences and Technology, Xidian University, Xi'an, China

J. Tian (✉)
CAS Key Laboratory of Molecular Imaging, Institute of Automation, Beijing, China
e-mail: jie.tian@ia.ac.cn

© Springer Nature Singapore Pte Ltd. 2018

J. Tian (ed.), *Multi-Modality Neuroimaging Study on Neurobiological Mechanisms of Acupuncture*, DOI 10.1007/978-981-10-4914-9_1

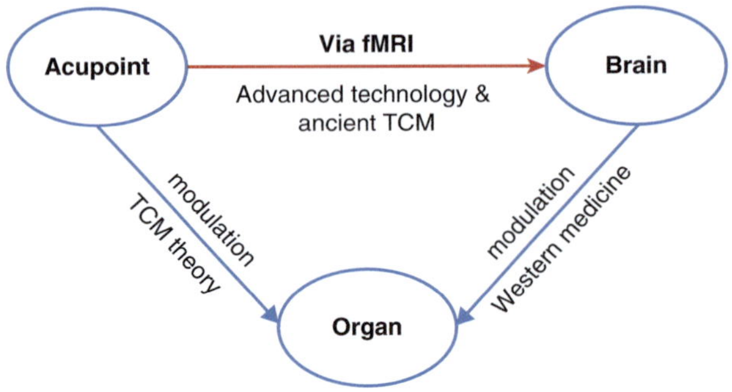

Fig. 1.1 Conceptual relationship between the acupoint, organ, and brain. The acupuncture effect can be evaluated via functional magnetic resonance imaging (fMRI). *TCM* traditional Chinese medicine

and acupoints (Cho et al. 1998). The inherent connectivity between the brain and various organs, and the classical view of TCM that considers a relationship between specific acupoints and organs, gives rise to an important question: what is the relationship between the brain and specific acupoints? Functional magnetic resonance imaging (fMRI) has been applied to explore relationships between acupuncture stimulation and functional areas of the brain cortex (Fig. 1.1), and this knowledge has opened a new window for researchers to investigate the central mechanisms of acupuncture. Here, we will provide a brief overview of fMRI principles and early fMRI studies evaluating the relationship between acupuncture and the brain. Chapter 2 will elaborate on these findings and on the ways in which fMRI can be used in the context of acupuncture research.

1.2 Principles of fMRI

Functional MRI is a noninvasive and relatively safe technique for the measurement and mapping of brain activity. fMRI is widely applied for the study of the brain and functional disruptions in the brain during pathological disease states.

1.2.1 MRI Contrast

MRI image acquisition relies on the use of a contrast agent. Different tissue characteristics can be visualized with the use of radiofrequency or gradient pulses and variations in the timing of image acquisition. The utility of contrast use in MRI derives from the decay of nuclear magnetization in a process called relaxation; the evaluation of differences in signal decay is specified by a given sequence “relaxation time.” There are three relaxation times that are of primary interest in MRI: T1, T2, and T2*. The T1 constant measures longitudinal relaxation time in the direction of the static magnetic field (B0). The T2 constant measures the transverse relaxation time in the plane perpendicular to the B0 field and notably is affected by molecular interactions and variations in B0. The T2 relaxation process is also affected by the combined time constant T2* (T2 star). T2* is the most relevant relaxation time for the study of the brain using contrast fMRI images (Matthews and Jezzard 2004).

1.2.1.1 Blood-Oxygen-Level-Dependent (BOLD) Contrast

BOLD contrast is employed in most fMRI studies. This method is based on the concept that neural activity affects the relative concentrations of oxygenated and deoxygenated hemoglobin in the local blood supply. Deoxyhemoglobin (dHb) is paramagnetic and therefore alters the MRI signal, while oxyhemoglobin (HbO_2) is diamagnetic and has no effect on the MRI signal. To this end, increases in dHb decrease the T2* constant, such that BOLD contrast represents the difference in T2* signal between HbO_2 and dHb (Fig. 1.2) (Yassa 2005; Chen and Glover 2015).

The principle underlying BOLD signal changes in response to brain activity is as follows. After stimulation, neural activation induces the absorption of oxygen from the local blood supply. In theory, this increase in paramagnetic dHb leads to the enhancement of field non-homogeneities and the reduction of BOLD signal. However, increased dHb is also accompanied by a surge in cerebral blood flow to increase the local supply of oxygenated blood and compensate for local deoxygenation. In this case, both the cerebral blood volume and hemoglobin oxygenation increase, and susceptibility-related dephasing decreases, which increases T2* signal and in turn enhances BOLD contrast (Yassa 2005).

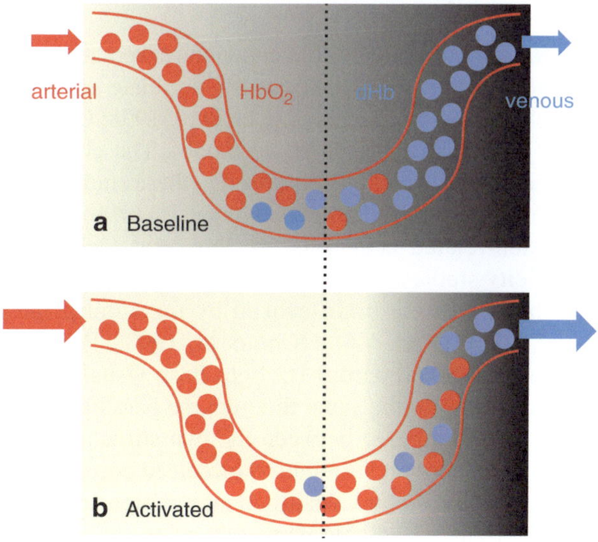

Fig. 1.2 Changes of HbO_2 and dHb concentrations between the baseline state (**a**) and the activated state (**b**) (Reprint with permission from Chen and Glover 2015)

1.2.1.2 Neural Basis of BOLD Signal and Neurovascular Coupling

The neuronal processes underlying changes in BOLD signal are related to synaptic inputs in active regions rather than the output level of neurons receiving synaptic inputs. This means that while BOLD signal on fMRI can reflect the synaptic activity that drives neuronal network communication, the information content of the activity is unknown.

Activity in the brain is tightly coupled to local blood flow. To this end, it is known that changes in the metabolic load are directly coupled to synaptic activation. One mechanism coupling vascular responses to synaptic activation involves the synaptic release of glutamate and subsequent Ca^{2+} alterations in neighboring astrocytes, which lead to the release of vasodilatory molecules. Accordingly, fMRI signals can be applied to explore functional responses in the brain using BOLD signals as a surrogate of synaptic activity (Seiji and Yul-Wan 2007).

1.3 Acupoint Specificity on fMRI

Acupoints are designated according to their functional and locational specificity. The concept of functional specificity purports that stimulation of a given acupoint causes corresponding changes in the BOLD signal in specific brain areas based on the function of the acupoint. Alternatively, locational specificity compares brain responses between a given acupoint and a sham acupoint (non-meridian or non-acupoint locations) or two different acupoints.

1.3.1 Acupoint Functional Specificity on fMRI

The earliest fMRI studies of acupuncture were focused on acupoint functional specificity and accordingly attempted to correlate acupoint stimulation with the activation of specific brain regions (Cho et al. 1998; Gareus et al. 2002; Siedentopf et al. 2002; Wu et al. 2002; Li et al. 2003b). The classic BLOCK experimental model original from psychology was used in these studies (Fig. 1.3). However, the conclusions of these studies have been inconsistent.

Vision-related acupoints are the most well-studied acupoints in functional specificity studies. Cho and colleagues first applied fMRI to evaluate BOLD signal changes in the brain evoked by the stimulation of vision-related acupoints BL67–BL60 (VA1–VA8) (Cho et al. 1998). Participants were subjected to conventional checkerboard 8-Hz light flash visual stimulation or acupoints stimulation according to the same time-course paradigm, and BOLD signal in the visual cortex was compared between the two stimulation methods. The results showed that visual acupoint stimulation produced cortical activation patterns very similar to those produced by visual light stimulation and that stimulation of BL67 in particular produced notable activation of the visual cortex. In a subsequent study, laser acupuncture and electroacupuncture (EA) were used to stimulate BL67

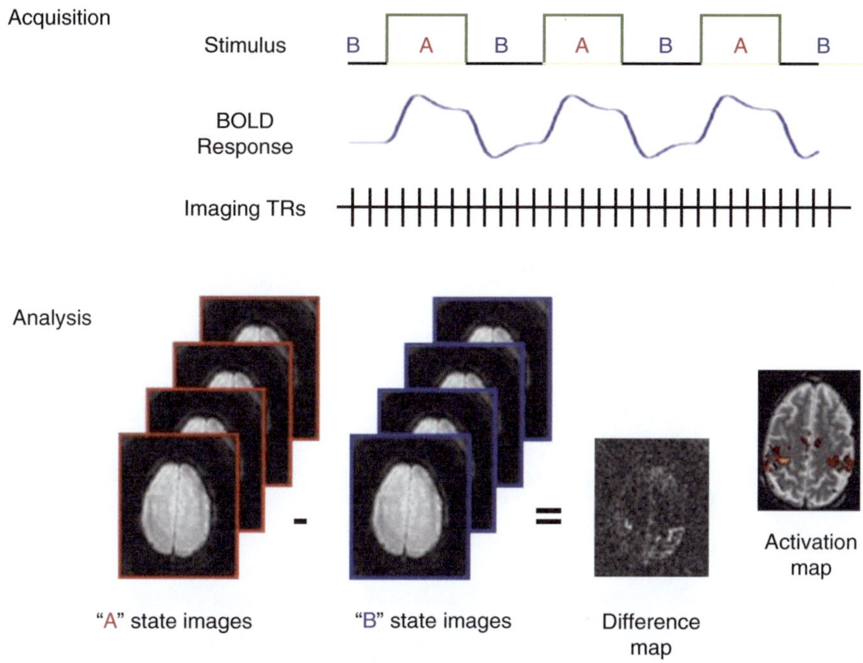

Fig. 1.3 The experimental model of early acupuncture fMRI studies. "A" is needle twirling state and "B" is needle retaining state (Reprint with permission from Chen and Glover 2015)

(Siedentopf et al. 2002; Li et al. 2003b), and the results confirmed the ability of acupoint stimulation to modulate the activity of visual brain areas.

In contrast, another research has refuted the ability of acupoint stimulation to produce activation in vision-related brain areas. Gareus and colleagues studied another vision-related acupoint, GB37, and compared acupuncture stimulation with visual stimulation using fMRI (Gareus et al. 2002). The recruited subjects were randomly divided into three groups and separately received visual stimulation and acupuncture stimulation without twisting the needle to avoid deqi, visual stimulation and acupuncture stimulation with deqi, or only acupuncture stimulation with deqi. The results demonstrated that activation of the visual cortex was only observed in subjects that received visual stimulation, whereas acupuncture stimulation had little impact on changes in BOLD signal in the visual cortex. Moreover, no activation of the visual cortex was detected in subjects that received acupuncture stimulation only (Fig. 1.4). Wu et al. also concluded that activation of the visual cortex was not a specific effect of vision-related acupoints (Wu et al. 2002). Soon after the publication of this study in 2006, Cho and colleagues retracted their functional specificity study on vision-related acupoint stimulation (Cho et al. 2006). In spite of this, the block design model was retained as a standard stimulation paradigm for fMRI studies of acupuncture.

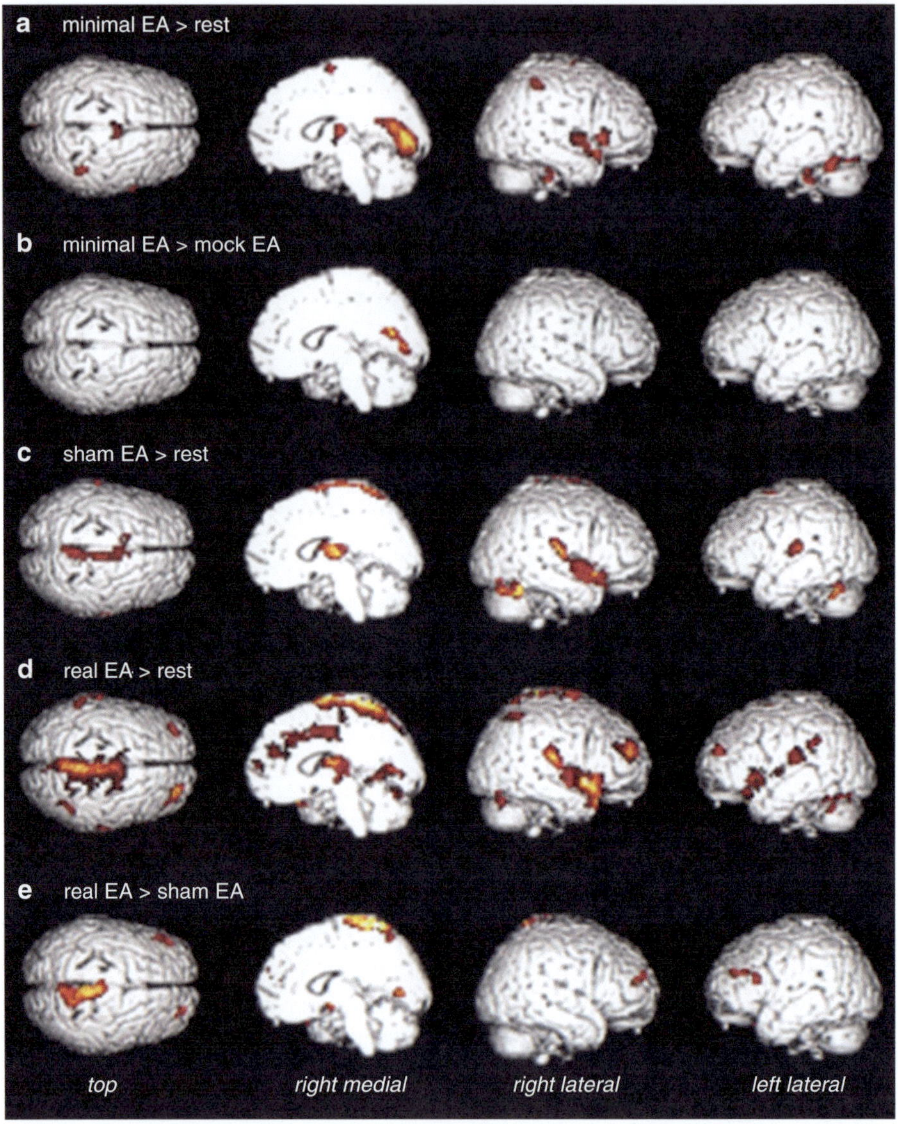

Fig. 1.4 Surface-rendered brain activation evoked by minimal, mock, sham, and real electroacupuncture (EA) stimulation (Reprint with permission from Wu et al. 2002). Minimal EA (**a**, **b**), sham EA (**c**), and real EA (**d**) all activated the medial occipital cortex (visual cortex). Real EA showed activations in the right medial occipital cortex, primary somatosensory-motor cortex, and hypothalamus and bilateral prefrontal cortex when comparing with sham EA (**e**)

An fMRI study was also used to evaluate brain responses to language-related acupoint stimulation (Li et al. 2003a). The results showed that, whereas word generation produced significant activation in the bilateral inferior frontal gyrus (IFG) and left superior temporal gyrus (STG), stimulation of two language-related acupoints (SJ8 and Du15) resulted in significant activation of the right IFG and bilateral STG.

The acupoint GB34, which is known to be a useful stimulation point for facilitating motor recovery after stroke, was investigated to determine its relationship with sensorimotor area activation (Jeun et al. 2005). Block design acupuncture stimulation at GB34 produced associated changes in the BOLD signal in bilateral sensorimotor areas, leading the authors to suggest that acupuncture-induced activation of sensorimotor areas may serve as a basis for the motor effects of GB34 stimulation.

Acupuncture has also been reported to increase salivary flow in healthy volunteers and patients with xerostomia (dry mouth) (Dawidson et al. 1997; Morganstein 2005). The neural substrates of this effect were explored using fMRI (Deng et al. 2008). LI2, a point commonly used for the clinical treatment of xerostomia, was selected as a target acupoint, and both BOLD signals and saliva production were measured before and after acupuncture manipulation. Deng and colleagues found that LI2 stimulation primarily produced activation in the bilateral insula and adjacent operculum, and moreover BOLD signal changes were associated with increased saliva production. Accordingly, the efficacy of LI2 stimulation was hypothesized to be related to its ability to produce insular activation.

LI4 is an effective acupoint for the treatment of facial palsy and facial muscle spasms (Xu et al. 2013). In the work by Xu et al., electroacupuncture at L14 produced typical signal deactivation in the bilateral hippocampus, parahippocampal gyrus, amygdala, anterior cingulate cortex (ACC), prefrontal lobe, and occipital lobe. Furthermore, Wang and colleagues found that activation of the precentral gyrus, which represents the movement of orofacial muscles, and cerebellum was related to the therapeutic effects of L14 in facial palsy and facial muscle spasm (Wang et al. 2007). Further studies are necessary to clarify whether these activation patterns represent functionally specific responses to acupoint stimulation or simply correlate with general somatosensory stimulation coupled to acupuncture.

1.3.2 Acupoint Locational Specificity on fMRI

In locational specificity studies, sham acupuncture is usually used as a control to exclude simple placebo effects. Several kinds of sham acupuncture strategies are used in research, including needling at a sham acupoint (Napadow et al. 2009a; Xiong et al. 2012), noninvasive placebo stimulation (e.g., Von Frey filament or Streitberger needle stimulation) at an acupoint site or sham acupoint site (Witt et al. 2005; Brinkhaus et al. 2013), and superficial needling at an acupoint site or sham acupoint site (Huang et al. 2005; Yin et al. 2010). Accordingly, both sham acupoints and sham stimulation have been used in acupuncture fMRI studies.

In 2010, Hui and colleagues hypothesized that acupuncture stimulation could evoke deactivation of the limbic-paralimbic-neocortical network (Hui et al. 2010a, b). This hypothesis was based on the observation that needling at LI4 or ST36 produced prominent deactivation in the nucleus accumbens, amygdala, hippocampus, parahippocampus, hypothalamus, ventral tegmental area, ACC, caudate, temporal

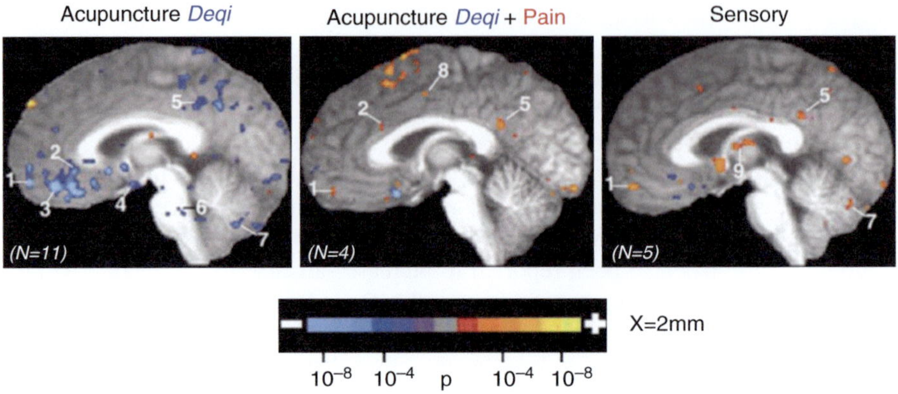

Fig. 1.5 The influence of subjective sensations on fMRI signal changes in the brain during acupuncture (or control stimulation) at ST36 (Reprint with permission from Hui et al. 2005). Regions: *1* frontal pole, *2* subgenual anterior cingulate, *3* ventromedial prefrontal cortex, *4* hypothalamus, *5* posterior cingulate cortex, *6* reticular formation, *7* cerebellar vermis, *8* middle cingulate, and *9* thalamus

pole, and insula, whereas needling produced activation in the somatosensory cortex in subjects who experienced deqi. Additionally, deactivation of the cerebellum was also noted during ST36 stimulation. Given that no decreases in signal were observed in subcortical structures in a superficial tactile stimulation control group, it was concluded that activity of the cerebro-cerebellar and limbic systems evoked by acupuncture needle manipulation might be a typical modulation effect of acupuncture (Fig. 1.5) (Wu et al. 1999; Hui et al. 2000, 2005). In a subsequent study by Fang et al., BOLD signal changes in response to manual acupuncture at LV3, LV2, and ST44 were investigated, and the results again demonstrated extensive deactivation of the limbic-paralimbic-neocortical network (Fang et al. 2009). Electroacupuncture at GB34, CV4, and CV12 has also been reported to modulate the activity of the limbic system (Wu et al. 2002; Fang et al. 2012). Functional connectivity of limbic-paralimbic-neocortical network was also explored during acupuncture versus tactile stimulation in a 2009 study by Hui and colleagues, and similar results were obtained (Hui et al. 2009). These studies all provided support for the hypothesis of Hui and colleagues that the deactivation of the limbic-paralimbic-neocortical network produced by acupuncture stimulation with deqi sensations might be the fundamental of acupuncture effect on various diseases.

Another research has challenged the hypothesis of Hui and colleagues. One review article found that BOLD responses associated with deqi were primarily characterized by activation rather than deactivation (Sun et al. 2013). Indeed, high-quality studies reporting robust BOLD responses to acupuncture stimulation with deqi have mainly highlighted four basic systems: the somatosensory system, motor system, sensory integration system, and special senses (vision, hearing) (Fig. 1.6). The most commonly activated areas in these studies included the secondary somatosensory cortex (SII), insula, primary somatosensory cortex (SI), cerebellum,

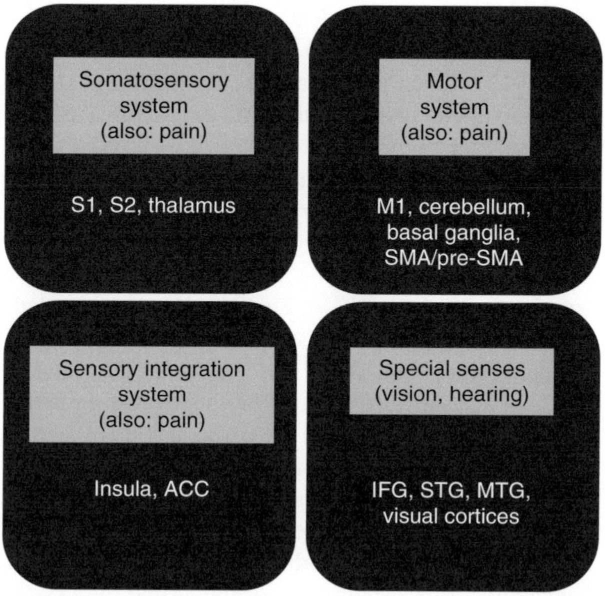

Fig. 1.6 Commonly reported areas of activation in fMRI studies of acupuncture (Reprint with permission from Beissner 2011)

thalamus, primary motor cortex, STG, visual cortex, IFG, premotor cortex, supplementary motor area (SMA), basal ganglia, medial temporal gyrus, and ACC (Beissner 2011). Moreover, Sun et al. suggested that extensive deactivation mediated by acupuncture on fMRI was a nonspecific pernicious consequence of global normalization (Sun et al. 2012a). Accordingly, the hypothesis of Hui et al. that acupuncture produces deactivation of the limbic-paralimbic-neocortical network has been largely rejected.

Regional changes in brain activity due to acupuncture have been explored in areas such as the cerebellum, periaqueductal gray (PAG), and default mode network (DMN). One acupuncture fMRI study compared acupoint, sham acupoint, and tactile stimulation conditions and found that acupuncture manipulation at PC6 specifically activated the cerebellum in the declive, nodulus, uvula of vermis, quadrangular lobule, cerebellar tonsil, and superior semilunar lobule of the cerebellum (Yoo et al. 2004). These alterations might be related to the clinical utility of PC6 for cerebellar vestibular modulation.

Both animal and human studies have demonstrated that the PAG is rich in opioid receptors and mediates analgesic effects via the descending inhibitory pathway of pain processing (Behbehani 1995; Linnman et al. 2012). A previous report by Napadow et al. used brainstem-focused cardiac-gated fMRI to show that longer duration (> 30 min) of electrostimulation at ST36 specifically modulated activity in the substantia nigra, nucleus raphe magnus, locus coeruleus, nucleus cuneiformis, and PAG (Napadow et al. 2009b). PAG activity was also shown to be modulated by needling at LI4 compared to needling at a sham acupoint (Liu et al. 2004). Further, the functional connectivity of the PAG was investigated after electrostimulation at LI4 and a sham acupoint, and it was found that LI4 stimulation specifically increased connectivity between the PAG, left posterior cingulate cortex (PCC), and precuneus and decreased connectivity between the PAG and right anterior insula (Zyloney et al. 2010). Taken together, these studies suggest that acupuncture may modulate brainstem nuclei including the PAG as part of its therapeutic effect, particularly with respect to pain perception.

DMN refers to the brain regions of deactivation during goal-directed tasks but activation during no task by using resting-state functional MRI (Andrews-Hanna et al. 2014). It has been suggested that the DMN instantiates processes that support emotional processing, self-referential mental activity, and the recollection of prior experiences (Raichle 2015). The DMN is also regarded as one of the most important networks for the pain connectome and is thought to play a significant role in persistent pain (Kucyi and Davis 2015). Researchers have attempted to demonstrate the effects of acupuncture on the DMN using resting fMRI data and heart rate variability (HRV) taken before and after true and sham acupuncture. In one study (Dhond et al. 2008), needling at PC6 produced increased DMN connectivity in areas including the ACC, PAG, amygdala, hippocampus, and middle temporal gyrus (MTG). Furthermore, the increased connectivity between DMN and hippocampus was associated with acupuncture-induced increases in parasympathetic tone and decreased sympathetic tone. Another study found that the DMN was subject to different patterns of modulation in response to stimulation at different acupoints or sham acupoints (Liu et al. 2009). Specifically, EA stimulation interrupted connectivity between the PCC and ACC and produced a negative interaction between the orbital prefrontal cortex (OFC) and left MTG. The ability of acupuncture to regulate connectivity within the DMN and enhance connectivity between the DMN and pain inhibitory, memory, and affective brain regional networks might contribute to acupuncture analgesia and other potential therapeutic effects.

The relationship between the autonomic nervous system (ANS) and brain activity during acupuncture was explored using cardiac-gated fMRI (Napadow et al. 2005a). The authors calculated the low frequency-to-high frequency (LF/HF) ratio from simultaneous HRV and used this index to express the activity of the ANS. EA at ST36 caused alterations in the LF/HF ratio that were significantly correlated with BOLD signal activities in the hypothalamus, dorsal raphe nucleus, PAG, and rostroventral medulla. Accordingly, acupuncture has demonstrated the ability to modulate activity in the ANS, and this feature may represent another component of its therapeutic effect.

1.3.3 Comparative Studies of Brain Responses to Acupoint Stimulation on fMRI

According to TCM, each acupoint has a particular location and function. An important question arises from this idea: what are the differences between different acupoints, and can these differences be visualized using fMRI? Acupoints in same meridian may have similar functions, whereas acupoints belonging to the same anatomical segment or existing adjacently have similar locations. Accordingly, new research has evaluated whether these acupoints also have shared neurological substrates. Whereas previous sections of this chapter described acupoint specificity, this next section will focus on studies differentiating between the effects of different acupoints.

Acupoints in the same meridian. The meridian is a concept of TCM that is defined as a pathway of qi and blood circulation. Accordingly, acupoints on the same meridian typically have similar functions. The acupoint pairs LR3/LR6 and ST36/ST43 were chosen to investigate brain responses to acupoints on the same meridian (Li et al. 2008). Stimulation at LR3 and LR6 both belonging to the liver meridian collectively activated the SI, superior parietal lobe (SPL), and cerebellum. Acupuncture at LR3 exclusively activated the medial frontal gyrus, middle frontal gyrus (MFG), MTG, ACC, lentiform nucleus, thalamus, and insula. In contrast, acupuncture at LR6 solely activated the ipsilateral superior frontal gyrus (SFG), middle occipital gyrus (MOG), and lingual gyrus. When stimulating at ST36 or ST43 which pertains to the stomach meridian, the SI, MFG, and cerebellum were the commonly activated regions. The SPL, MOG, and occipital pole were also activated by acupuncture at ST36. The active areas including in the SII, IFG, and thalamus were evoked only by acupuncture at ST43. However, this study lacked a statistical comparison between acupoint fMRI results and accordingly may not have been accurately reported. Another study reported partial overlap between brain activity changes in response to stimulation at PC6 and PC7, although PC6 produced a greater extent of cortical activation than did PC7 (Bai et al. 2010); only the posterior insula exhibited differential deactivation between the two acupoint stimulation conditions. Taken together, it can be concluded that while some overlap has been reported in brain responses to the stimulation of different acupoints in the same meridian, there exists no clear evidence to support the hypothesis that meridian acupoints exclusively produce the same brain responses.

Acupoints in the same nerve segment or anatomical location. Skin and tissue within a nerve segment share the same ascending sensory pathways. HT7 and SI6 are two acupoints located in the same nerve segment that were stimulated to investigate whether acupoints with similar locations elicit similar specific brain responses (Zhong et al. 2010). Acupuncture at HT7 increased BOLD signal in the right post-central gyrus and left IFG, whereas acupuncture at SI6 increased the signal in the left IPL and right IFG. Another study investigated the specific functional brain networks modulated by another pair of acupoints located in the same segment, GB40 and KI3 (Chen et al. 2012). Post-acupuncture resting-state functional brain network maps were constructed after needling at each acupoint. When comparing resting-state networks before and after KI3 stimulation, increased connectivities between the posttemporal cortex and dorsolateral PFC as well as the posttemporal cortex and ventromedial PFC were identified. These connectivities were related to cognitive functions, consistent with the known function of KI3. In contrast, increased connectivity between the anterior insula and temporal cortex emerged following acupuncture at GB40 relative to the resting state. The abovementioned studies demonstrate that stimulation at different acupoints in the same anatomical segment does not necessarily evoke similar brain responses; rather, specific responses appear to be related to the mechanism of the known therapeutic effects for each acupoint.

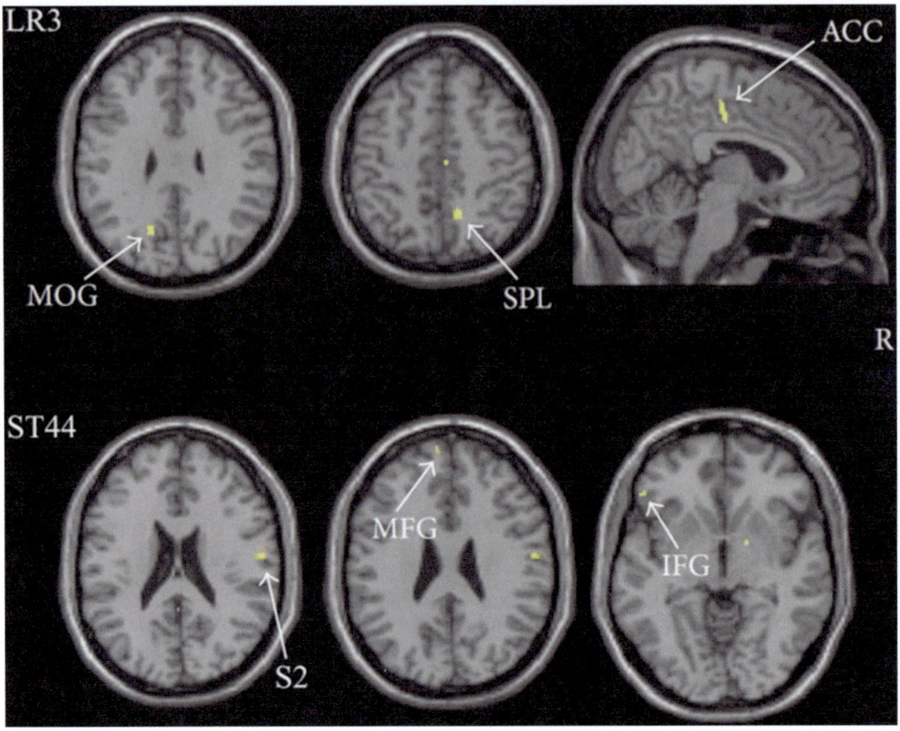

Fig. 1.7 Activation in response to LR3 and ST44 stimulation with respect to stimulation of a nearby non-acupoint (Reprint from Liu et al. 2013). *ACC* anterior cingulate cortex, *IFG* inferior frontal gyrus, *MFG* middle frontal gyrus, *MOG* middle occipital gyrus, *SII* secondary somatosensory area, *SPL* superior parietal lobe

Two adjacent acupoints, LR3 and ST44, and a nearby non-acupoint were selected to investigate relative specificity among different acupoints. Healthy volunteers were recruited and received acupuncture at one of the three points during image scanning. The results revealed that areas commonly activated by LR3 or ST44 stimulation were the contralateral SI and ipsilateral cerebellum. LR3-specific activation sites included the contralateral MOG, ipsilateral medial PFC, SPL, MTG, rostral ACC, lentiform nucleus, insula, and contralateral thalamus. In contrast, ST44-specific activation sites included the ipsilateral SII, contralateral MFG, IFG, lingual gyrus, lentiform nucleus, and bilateral PCC (Fig. 1.7) (Liu et al. 2013). Consistent with the abovementioned studies, Liu et al. demonstrated that stimulation at adjacent acupoints elicited distinct patterns of cerebral activation potentially related to the functional effects of each specific acupoint.

Specificities of acupoints in different meridians. According to TCM theory, it has also been proposed that some acupoints in different meridians might have similar functions. To this end, a few studies have evaluated the ability of acupoints with similar therapeutic effects to produce similar alterations in BOLD signal on fMRI (Fang et al. 2006; Zhong et al. 2010; Claunch et al. 2012). The specificity and commonality of brain responses to acupuncture at LI4, ST36, and LV3, which are acupoints used to treat pain disorders, were evaluated using fMRI (Claunch et al. 2012). Common activated areas included the SII, dorsolateral and dorsomedial PFC, anterior insula, and thalamus. However, differences were observed in the spatial distribution and degree of deactivation of the medial PFC, medial parietal cortex, and medial temporal lobe, suggesting that the three acupoints produced brain responses some relative specificity. Further supporting this point, while LI4 stimulation primarily elicited responses in the pregenual cingulate and hippocampus, ST36 elicited responses in the subgenual cingulate, and LV3 produced changes in the posterior hippocampus and posterior cingulate. Accordingly, these acupoints may modulate the same intrinsic global networks by different mechanisms to produce the same therapeutic effect. The commonality and specificity of brain responses to acupoints in different meridians have been similarly reported for other acupoints (Fang et al. 2006).

In summary, although the results of acupuncture fMRI studies are heterogeneous, multiple studies have demonstrated the ability of acupuncture to modulate activity within specific brain regions, including the somatosensory cortices, limbic system, basal ganglia, brain stem, and cerebellum (Huang et al. 2012). Moreover, several studies support the ability of acupoints to produce brain responses in a manner potentially representing the functional specificity of their therapeutic effects (Bai et al. 2010; Chen et al. 2012; Claunch et al. 2012; Liu et al. 2013). This idea is supported by the fact that acupoints located in the same meridian or in the same anatomical segment can produce different brain responses with relative specificity.

1.4 fMRI Studies of Acupuncture Sensation

Acupuncture sensation or deqi refers to the experience of soreness, numbness, fullness, heaviness, and so forth elicited by needle insertion at a certain depth at a given acupoint. At the same time, the operator may feel heaviness or tension around the needle (Hui et al. 2007; Kong et al. 2007a). Notably, deqi is distinguishable from sharp pain that can sometimes emerge during acupuncture needling, which is regarded as non-deqi and harmful (Hui et al. 2011). Deqi is considered to be an indispensable component of acupuncture treatment, and this idea is supported by several clinical studies (Berman et al. 2004; Witt et al. 2005; Xiong et al. 2012). An understanding of deqi is therefore essential for elucidating the mechanisms and neural substrates of acupuncture.

An fMRI study was conducted to determine neurological correlates of deqi and to determine how and why this sensation is connected to therapeutic outcome (Napadow et al. 2009a). Healthy volunteers were subjected to acupuncture stimulation at PC6 and asked to rate deqi sensation using a custom-built, MRI-compatible potentiometer. Non-insertive cutaneous stimulation was used as a sham control. Acupuncture induced stronger and more complex sensations with significant persistence after the cessation of needle manipulation, leading to more run-time spent rating low and moderate sensations, compared to sham control stimulation.

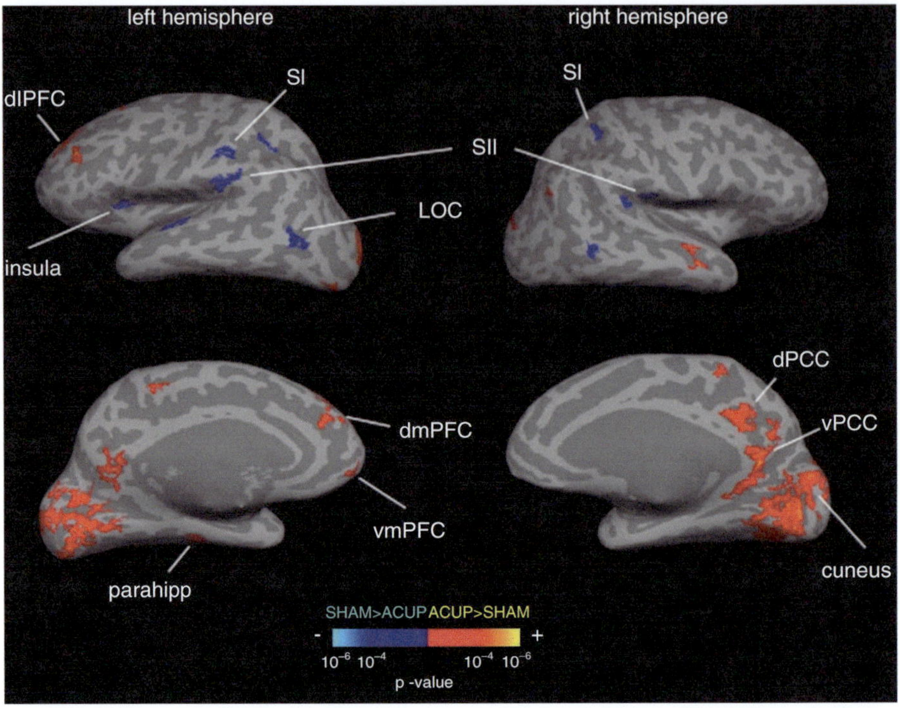

Fig. 1.8 Percept-related fMRI group difference maps (acupuncture simulation minus sham stimulation) (Reprint with permission from Napadow et al. 2009a)

Acupuncture sensation was moreover associated with activation in the SII, insula, and dorsomedial PFC and deactivation in DMN regions (the PCC and precuneus). In contrast, sham stimulation produced greater degrees of activation in the SI, SII, and insula and greater degrees of deactivation in DMN regions. The results of this study concluded that deqi sensation was specifically associated with increased activation of the anterior and posterior dorsomedial and dorsolateral PFC (Fig. 1.8). The ability of dorsomedial PFC activity to strengthen the top-down regulation of nociceptive input could potentially represent one mechanism of acupuncture analgesia.

Research has also compared the effects of deqi and acute pain sensations from needling using brain fMRI BOLD signal. In one study, fMRI images collected during stimulation at LI4 were classified into predominantly deqi sensation (deqi scores greater than pain sensation scores) and predominantly acute pain sensation (pain scores greater than deqi scores) (Asghar et al. 2010). Probabilistic masks of brain regions of interest in the limbic/subcortical structures (the insula, hippocampus, amygdala, thalamus, and posterior/anterior cingulate gyrus) and cerebellum were selected. A comparison of the results revealed that, during predominantly deqi sensation produced by superficial or deep needling, significant negative signals were observed bilaterally in the insula, hippocampus, amygdala, thalamus, and cerebellum (Fig. 1.9). In another

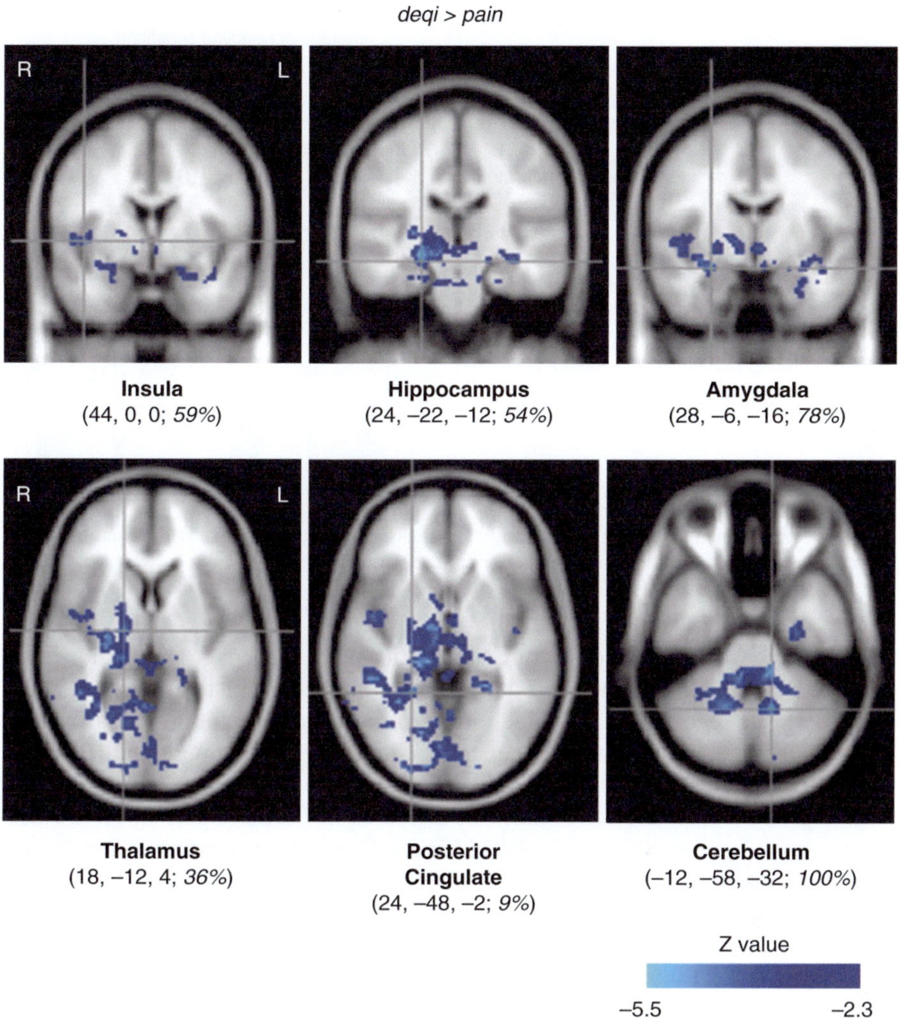

Fig. 1.9 Functional maps showing significant clusters for the deqi > pain condition for the selected regions of interest (Reprint with permission from Asghar et al. 2010)

study that compared pure deqi sensation (deqi without sharp pain) and mixed sensations (deqi with sharp pain) using fMRI, mixed sensations produced significantly stronger bilateral activation in the putamen, thalamus, and cerebellum (CrusI and CrusII) compared to pure deqi sensation during acupuncture stimulation at ST36 (Sun et al. 2012b). These studies suggest that patterns of BOLD responses to sharp pain or mixed sensation are partially distinguishable (in terms of spatial distribution) from those produced by deqi sensation. These studies moreover suggest that subjects who experience sharp pain or mixed sensation should be excluded or separated from the central population in future studies of acupuncture and deqi.

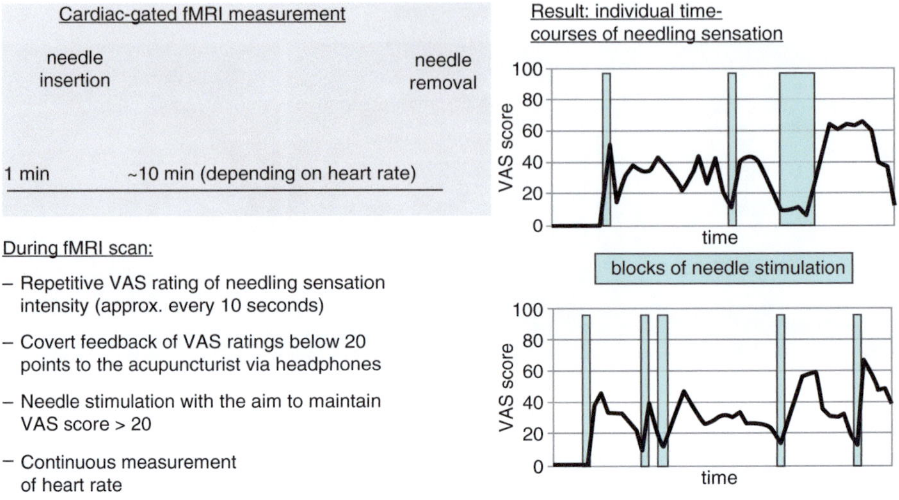

Fig. 1.10 Experimental design of the study by Beissner and colleagues. *VAS* visual analogue scale (Reprint with permission from Beissner et al. 2012)

Similarities between acupuncture stimulation and deep pain stimulation have also been explored. Beissner and colleagues combined brainstem-sensitive fMRI with heart rate recording and online ratings of needling sensation to measure and compare the neural correlates of acupuncture and deep pain stimulation (Beissner et al. 2012). The details of the experimental design are summarized in Fig. 1.10.

The group results showed significant increases in BOLD signal in the SI, SII, supramarginal gyrus, SPL, ACC, IFG/MFG/SFG, insula (extending to the frontal operculum and OFC), lateral occipital cortex, dorsolateral PFC, and locus coeruleus. Deactivation was observed in the ventromedial PFC/perigenual ACC. Heart rate changes during acupuncture stimulation at PC6 were concluded to be the consequence of a shift in sympatho-vagal balance toward vagal predominance, which might have been mediated by a circumscribed network of cortical and subcortical areas in the ventromedial PFC/perigenual ACC, dorsolateral PFC, locus coeruleus, hypothalamus, ventrolateral medulla, and nucleus ambiguus. Beissner and colleagues concluded that there were strong similarities in BOLD signal during acupuncture needling sensation versus deep pain stimulation. Moreover, acupuncture induced heart rate changes that were mediated by the same autonomic network (in the mesencephalic and brainstem nuclei) as that activated by deep pain stimulation. Based on these results, it can be hypothesized that acupuncture might represent a special type of deep pain stimulation; however, additional studies are required to investigate this possibility.

In a novel approach, Jin and colleagues used lidocaine anesthesia to investigate the effects of deqi (Jin et al. 2014). Volunteers were recruited to complete two fMRI scans: one during manual acupuncture at ST36 and another after the administration of local anesthesia and during manual acupuncture at the same acupoint. The bilateral SI,

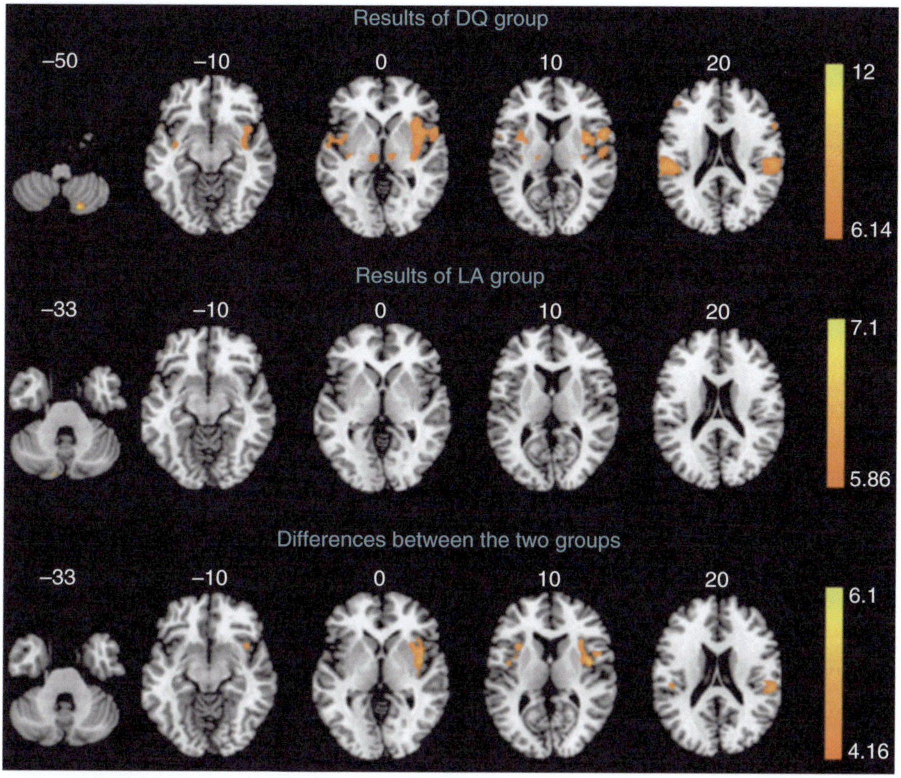

Fig. 1.11 BOLD responses for the deqi (DQ) group, local anesthesia (LA) group, and between-group differences (Reprint from Jin et al. 2014)

insula, ipsilateral IFG, IPL, claustrum, and contralateral ACC were remarkably activated by acupuncture at ST36 (Fig. 1.11); however, local anesthesia precluded a majority of deqi sensation and inhibited brain responses in these regions. The results of this study do not only assist the identification of deqi-related brain regions but also offer a potential non-deqi control condition for use in future studies.

In summary, studies have developed different perspectives of deqi and its neurological substrates using fMRI. The results of these studies are heterogeneous due to different research objectives, experimental designs, and control groups. Positive BOLD responses associated with deqi were primarily observed in cortical areas relevant to the processing of somatosensory or nociceptive information. Moreover, different brain responses were observed for pure deqi sensation versus mixed sensations. However, there were similarities between the BOLD response patterns evoked by acupuncture deqi sensation and deep pain sensation. A standardized method for characterizing and quantifying deqi will permit a deeper understanding of deqi and sharp pain sensations, allow the determination of a proper control condition for further research, and ultimately reveal the neural substrates of deqi and acupuncture mechanisms (Sun et al. 2013).

1.5 fMRI Studies of Acupuncture Manipulation

Various stimulation methods are used for clinical acupuncture treatment, including manual acupuncture (MA), EA, transcutaneous electrical stimulation, acupressure, and laser acupuncture. Furthermore, various parameters of acupuncture can be optimized for treatment including needling depth, needle retention time, and frequency. A number of fMRI studies have addressed differences between the effects of these techniques on brain responses.

1.5.1 fMRI Studies of Different Acupuncture Stimulation Modalities

MA is a traditional form of acupuncture that has been used clinically for thousands of years. In contrast, EA is a relatively new technique that advantageously allows the objective and quantifiable adjustment of stimulation frequency at a given acupoint. The brain activation patterns evoked by MA and EA were characterized in normal human subjects using fMRI (Kong et al. 2002). A continuous rectangular waveform and a frequency of 3 Hz were selected for EA stimulation of left LI4, while for MA, the needle was inserted and manually rotated clockwise and counterclockwise at an approximate rate of 180 times per minute (3 Hz). EA produced statistically greater BOLD signal increases than MA in the precentral gyrus, postcentral gyrus, insular cortex, and SFG. In another study comparing the central effects of tactile stimulation, MA, and EA at different frequencies (2 Hz and 100 Hz) at ST36 using fMRI, all forms of stimulation were noted to increase signal in the SII. Acupuncture but not tactile stimulation produced signal increases in the anterior insula and signal decreases in limbic and paralimbic structures including the amygdala, anterior hippocampus, subgenual cortex, retrosplenial cingulate cortex, ventromedial PFC, frontal pole, and temporal pole. Similar to the abovementioned study, another study also demonstrated that EA (particularly at a low frequency) produced more widespread brain activation than MA (Napadow et al. 2005b). These results suggested that EA and MA might recruit different brain mechanisms in the exertion of their therapeutic effects.

Transcutaneous electrical acupoint stimulation (TEAS) is a simple, noninvasive method that has been popularized in clinical and domestic settings. One study used resting-state fMRI to investigate alterations in the DMN and sensorimotor network (SMN) after MA, EA, and TEAS (Jiang et al. 2013). Changes in connectivity after MA and EA primarily involved the DMN: after MA, increased connectivity was observed in the precuneus, MOG, temporal gyrus, and premotor cortex, while decreased connectivity was found in the STG. EA produced increased connectivity in the MOG, fusiform gyrus, and cerebellum, while decreased connectivity was observed in the IPL and cuneus. By contrast, TEAS generally increased connectivity in the SMN in areas including the SI, premotor cortex, dorsal ACC, SMA, superior temporal lobe, and parietal lobe (Fig. 1.12).

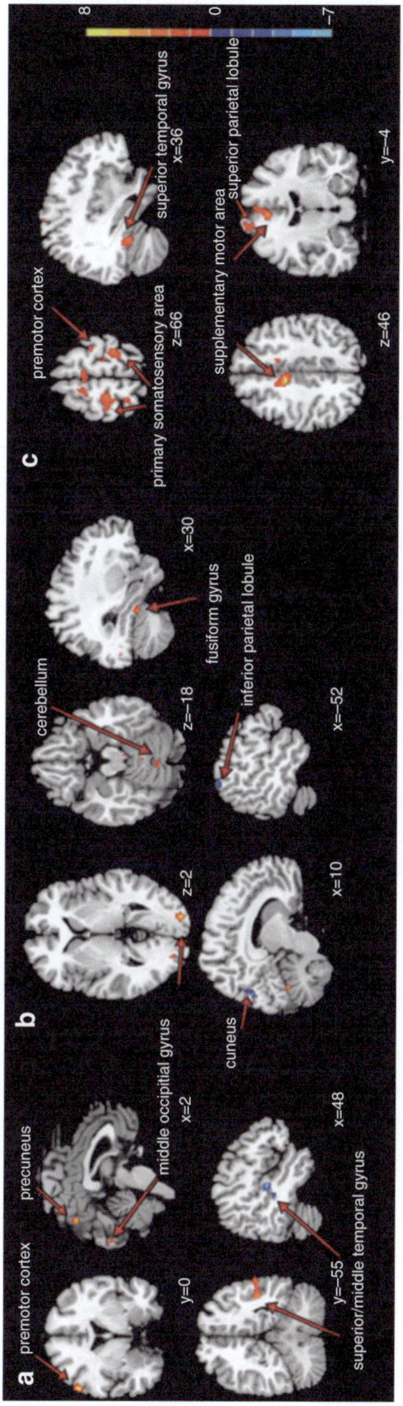

Fig. 1.12 Changes in functional connectivity in the default mode network and sensorimotor network following manual acupuncture (Reprint from Jiang et al. 2013) (**a**), electroacupuncture (**b**), or transcutaneous electrical acupoint stimulation (**c**)

Acupressure is an alternative technique that is similar in principle to acupuncture but aims to clear blockages in affected meridians using tactile pressure stimulation. Differences in brain responses to acupressure versus acupuncture at the same acupoint have been assessed using fMRI. Cho and colleagues performed acupressure and acupuncture stimulation at left LI11 and ST36 and evaluated differences in brain activation on fMRI (Cho et al. 2010). In comparison to left LI11 acupressure, acupuncture stimulation produced greater degrees of activation in the bilateral parahippocampal gyrus, cerebellum, left thalamus, and right PCC. Alternatively, in comparison to left ST36 acupressure, acupuncture enhanced activation in the secondary motor cortex, ACC, PCC, primary visual cortex, pons, and medulla. It was concluded that acupuncture produced greater activation in a larger number of regions, especially in the limbic system, than acupressure alone at the same acupoint.

Laser acupuncture refers to the use of low-energy laser light as a substitute for traditional acupuncture needling to influence the flow of current at acupuncture points. It has been previously reported that laser acupuncture is an effective treatment for myofascial pain, postoperative nausea and vomiting, and chronic tension headache (Baxter et al. 2008). The differential effects of laser acupuncture and manual needle acupuncture have also been evaluated using fMRI. LR8, which is a valid acupuncture point for depression, was stimulated using both laser and manual needle acupuncture in healthy participants. Needle acupuncture produced greater activation in the left precentral gyrus whereas laser acupuncture evoked greater activation in the left precuneus (Quah-Smith et al. 2013).

The abovementioned studies lead to the perspective that different acupuncture modalities induce different patterns of brain activation. On this premise, it can be hypothesized that the underlying therapeutic mechanisms of action for each modality may be distinct from one another. Future comparative studies are required to determine the neurological substrates of each modality and their therapeutic utilities in different contexts.

1.5.2 Influence of Acupuncture Parameters on Evoked Brain Responses

Differences between superficial and deep acupuncture needling were explored using fMRI in a study by MacPherson and colleagues (MacPherson et al. 2008). Two fMRI scans were taken in random order in a block design during superficial and deep needling at right LI4. The study demonstrated that there were no significant differences in BOLD signal responses, suggesting that neural responses to acupuncture at LI4 do not vary according to the depth of needling stimulation. This data is consistent with the view that Japanese and Chinese styles of acupuncture, which utilize superficial and deep needling techniques, respectively, offer equivalent therapeutic effects.

TCM proposes that the duration of acupuncture needling influences the resultant therapeutic effect. One study investigated brain responses to different durations of needling at LI4 using fMRI (Li et al. 2006). Acupuncture was performed at right LI4 for 30, 60, or 180 s. The results showed that longer durations of manual acupuncture induced the activation of more therapeutically significant areas. Common areas of activation among the three conditions included the bilateral transverse temporal gyrus, left SII, right IPL, and cerebellum (posterior lobe); whereas common areas of deactivation included the bilateral orbital gyrus, anterior inferior temporal gyrus (ITG), and bilateral occipital lobe. Pairwise comparisons were as follows: comparing 60-s stimulation to 30-s stimulation, deactivation was observed in the bilateral orbital gyrus, right anterior temporal lobe, and pons, whereas activation was observed in the right anterior IFG and ITG. Comparing 180-s stimulation to either 30-s or 60-s stimulation, deactivation was observed in the bilateral dorsolateral PFC and a small region of the MFG, whereas activation was observed in the bilateral temporal pole, cerebellum, and occipital lobe. The ability of acupuncture stimulation to produce different brain responses according to the duration of stimulation provides useful insight for clinical application. However, tolerance-like effects have also been observed in response to repeated stimulation at BL62 (Yeo et al. 2010), suggesting that future studies should carefully optimize both the duration and frequency of acupuncture simulation in order to maximize its therapeutic effects.

1.6 fMRI Studies of Acupuncture Analgesia

As mentioned throughout this first chapter, a number of studies have demonstrated the efficacy of acupuncture analgesia in both experimental models of pain and clinical chronic pain (Lin and Chen 2009; Leung 2012; Han 2011). Animal studies suggest that central opioid receptors are important for mediating the analgesic effects of acupuncture (Han 2011). The accumulated fMRI studies also support the idea that the central nervous system plays a role in the treatment effects of acupuncture for pain (He et al. 2015; Scheffold et al. 2015). Here, we will provide a brief introduction to acupuncture analgesia that will be further elaborated in the subsequent chapter.

Zhang et al. investigated the relationship between brain network activation and the analgesic effects of EA stimulation using fMRI (Zhang et al. 2003). Low (2 Hz) and high (100 Hz) frequency EA stimulation in addition to minimal EA at ST36 and SP6 were randomly performed in a block design on healthy volunteers. Analgesic effects were measured in a separate session 1–7 days after fMRI scanning. Individual pain thresholds were determined by timing the latency of withdrawal from a noxious thermal stimulus administered to the dorsum of the foot, and increased averaged latencies after EA were calculated as percentages to represent the analgesic effects of EA. Common areas of fMRI activation between the two stimulation frequencies included the bilateral SII and insula; moreover, activations of the contralateral ACC and thalamus were positively correlated with analgesic effect. In the 2 Hz EA group, positive correlations were observed between analgesic effect and activation in the contralateral primary motor area, SMA, and ipsilateral STG; and a

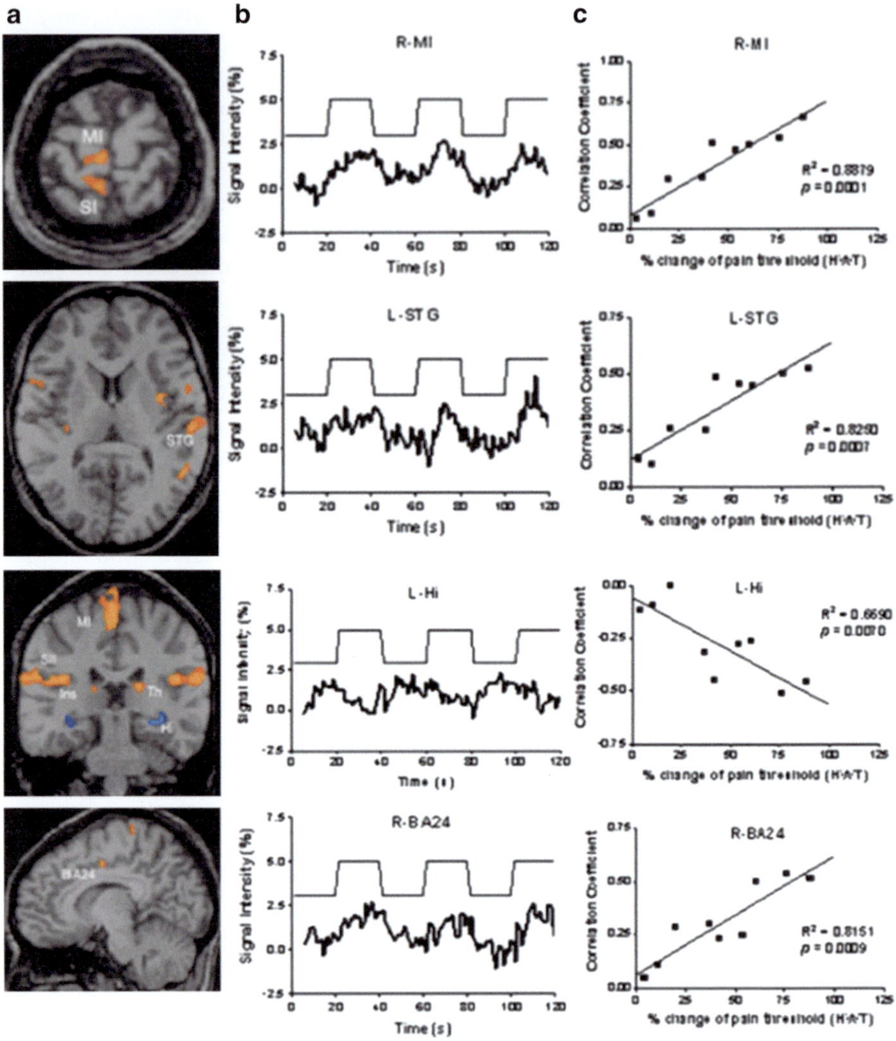

Fig. 1.13 Functional imaging data after 2-Hz electroacupuncture stimulation (Reprint with permission from Zhang et al. 2003)

negative correlation was found between analgesic effect and activation in the bilateral hippocampus (Fig. 1.13). In the 100 Hz EA group, positive correlations between analgesic effect and activation were observed in the contralateral IPL, ipsilateral ACC, nucleus accumbens, and pons, while a negative correlation was found between analgesic effect and activation in the contralateral amygdala (Fig. 1.14). The results suggest that different frequencies of EA stimulation may modulate different brain networks to produce analgesic effects. To this end, Jiang and colleagues similarly found that different frequencies of TEAS produced experimental relief from acute

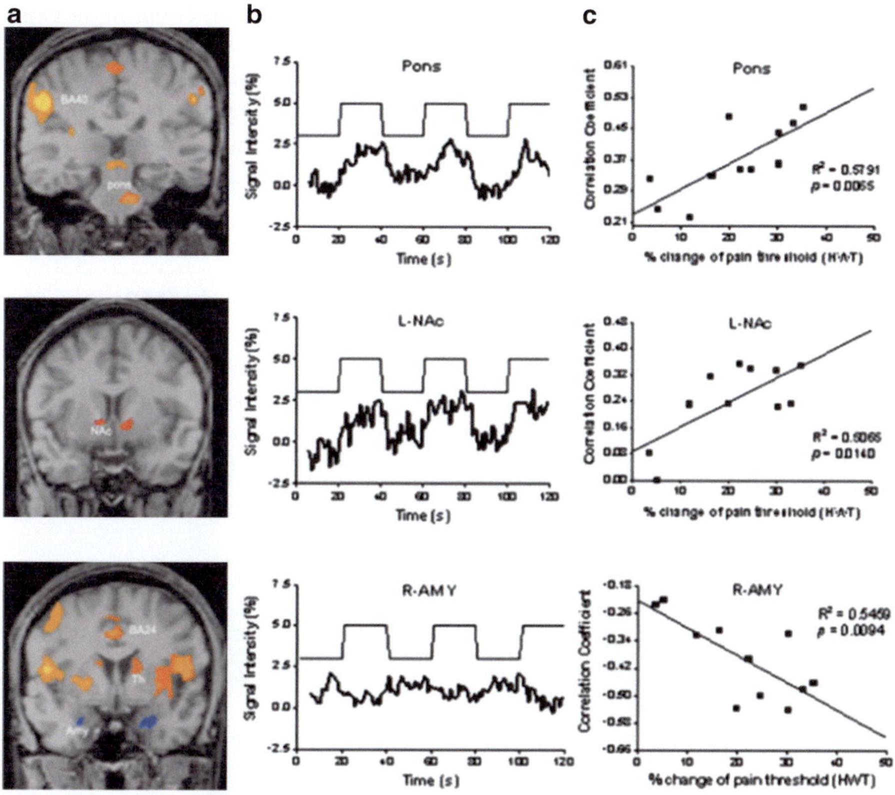

Fig. 1.14 Functional imaging data after 100-Hz electroacupuncture stimulation (Reprint with permission from Zhang et al. 2003)

pain induced by potassium iontophoresis in a manner that was partially overlapping but distinctly represented on fMRI (Jiang et al. 2014).

It is well known that expectation can significantly alter pain perception and responses (Atlas and Wager 2012; Elsenbruch 2014). The interaction between expectation and acupuncture analgesia was previously investigated by Kong and colleagues using fMRI (Kong et al. 2009a, b). The results showed that, although subjects in both the high- and low-expectancy groups experienced comparable magnitudes of acupuncture sensations in response to EA, analgesic effects were significantly different and expressly modulated by expectancy. Positive expectation may therefore enhance acupuncture analgesia. With regard to the neurological basis of this effect, fMRI signal in the high-expectancy group showed corresponding decreases in the bilateral rostral ACC/MPFC, left OFC, and dorsolateral PFC during application of a noxious stimulus. Moreover, while true and sham acupuncture produced equal magnitudes of subjective analgesia in the high-expectancy group, the fMRI analysis showed that true acupuncture was associated with greater decreases in activation of the left insula, putamen, claustrum, STG, and IFG during noxious stimulus application compared to the sham group.

In conclusion, the underlying mechanisms of acupuncture analgesia and expectancy-evoked placebo analgesia appear to be mediated by different neurological mechanisms or associated with different patterns of brain activity. The brain network related to acupuncture analgesia might therefore be altered on the basis of emotional status (high versus low expectancy).

1.7 Methodological and Statistical Issues in Early fMRI Studies of Acupuncture

A review by Beissner and Henke characterized the ways in which many early acupuncture fMRI studies failed to adopt the methodological standards applied to most other fMRI investigations (Fig. 1.15) (Beissner and Henke 2011). These issues are

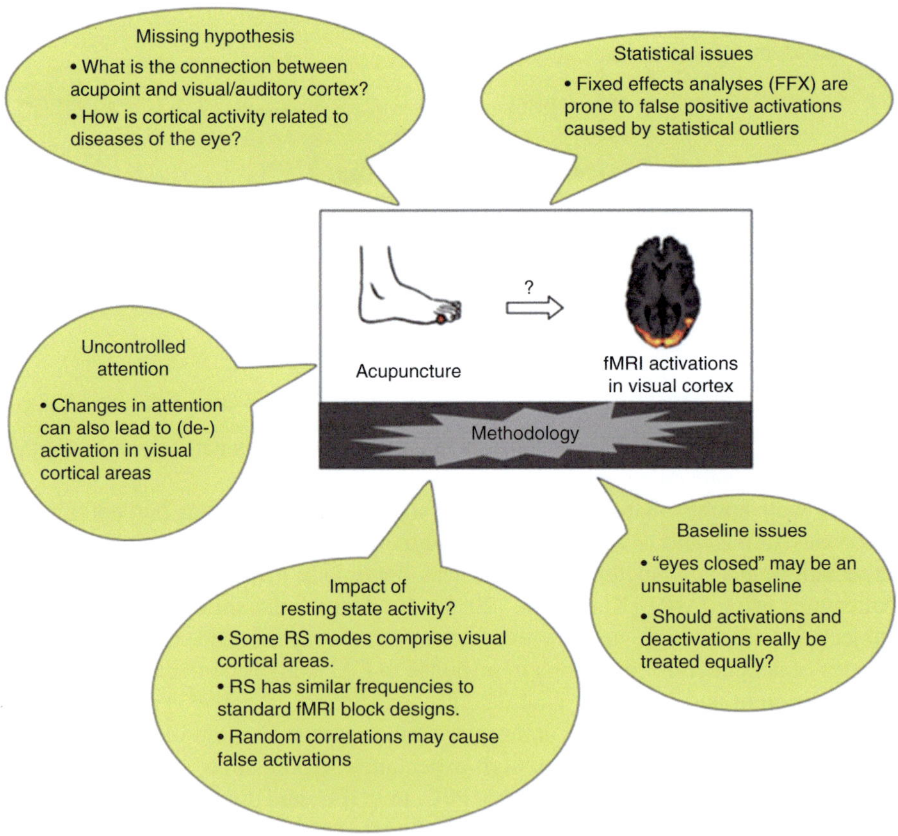

Fig. 1.15 Alternative explanations for the observed activation of visual cortical areas in early acupuncture fMRI studies (Reprint from Beissner and Henke 2011)

thought to be a primary source of heterogeneity in the research findings reported in this chapter. The goal of this section is to review and discuss these methodological issues and to present several reasonable suggestions for future research conduct and interpretation.

Subject recruitment and selection. An important characteristic of acupuncture according to TCM is its bidirectional regulatory effects in unhealthy individuals. In early acupuncture fMRI studies, most studies selected healthy volunteers as research subjects to explore the central therapeutic mechanisms of acupuncture (Huang et al. 2012). However, whether these studies failed to observe the state-dependent nature of acupuncture effects is unclear. Thus, it may be important and more appropriate to investigate the mechanisms of acupuncture therapy in patients with indications for acupuncture, as is the trend in recent research. Additionally, it is important that the criteria applied for patient inclusion in acupuncture studies strictly adhere to those applied in similar trials of drug efficacy for the same or similar indications.

Response pattern assumptions. Initially, fMRI was used to confirm and explore basic questions in experimental psychology and cognitive neuroscience using one of two experimental designs: a block design or an event-related design. The same designs, especially the block design, were applied in early acupuncture fMRI studies (Wu et al. 1999, 2002; Hui et al. 2000, 2005; Li et al. 2003a, b). However, the block design was used based on the hypothesis that brain-responsive regions could quickly enter into a non-resting state, remain stable during a given stimulus, and efficiently revert to the resting state after stimulus removal. This hypothesis is not compatible with the observation that acupuncture can have sustained modulatory effects. On this premise, the use of a block design may have been inappropriate in fMRI studies of acupuncture, and the reported responses may have represented immediate sensations resultant from needle manipulation and accompanying emotions, as well as the central processing of attention and cognition. As an alternative, resting-state fMRI is an attractive new research method that may be more appropriate for investigating the sustained effects of acupuncture.

Group analysis methods. Different acupuncture studies have employed diverse strategies for group analyses. In general, there are four categories of group analyses: (1) non-model methodology, which simply calculates the averages and frequencies of data for different subjects (Cho et al. 1998); (2) fixed effects model methodology, which is a statistical model that represents the observed quantities in terms of explanatory variables that are treated as if the quantities were nonrandom (Siedentopf et al. 2002); (3) random effects model methodology, which assumes that an individual specific effect is unrelated to independent variables (Kong et al. 2007b); and (4) mixed effects model methodology, which is based on the assumption of both intersubject and between-group differences (Zhang et al. 2016). Although the non-model and fixed effect model methodologies have been largely eliminated from mainstream fMRI studies, a majority of early acupuncture fMRI studies used these models (particularly the fixed effects model); only recently has acupuncture research begun the transition to use of a random effects model for group analyses (Beissner and Henke 2011). Additional studies using random effects and mixed effects models are required in order to enrich the field of acupuncture research with more methodologically sound and reproducible data.

Statistical powers. Apart from rational analysis methods, an appropriate threshold for significance is one of the most important aspects for guaranteeing result reliability. Numerous review articles (Bennett et al. 2009; Poldrack 2012; Eklund et al. 2016) have offered discussions specifically addressing threshold corrections in fMRI studies and have repeatedly stressed that multiple contrasts and corrections for thresholds have no reason or possibility for compromise, given that uncorrected thresholds do not inform result reliability under any circumstance. Although the random effects model has recently risen in popularity for group analyses in fMRI-based studies, existing acupuncture fMRI studies using random effects models have mostly adopted an uncorrected threshold of $p < 0.001$ (Beissner 2011). These thresholds were argued to be invalid by the aforementioned review articles. Therefore, there exists an urgent need for fMRI studies employing corrected, appropriate thresholds in the field of acupuncture research.

Sample size. Theoretically speaking, population characteristics are best represented by larger sample sizes. Indeed, researchers have proposed that large sample sizes and rigidly corrected thresholds are indispensable in fMRI studies (Poldrack 2012). Yet, most early acupuncture fMRI studies were based on smaller samples that made it difficult to adopt a rigidly corrected threshold (Beissner 2011). This confounding issue is an important point of consideration when interpreting the results of early acupuncture fMRI studies.

Result interpretation. Many fMRI-based cognitive investigations have identified significant deactivation patterns and correctly interpreted them with relative caution. Most of these deactivations were reported in the DMN and presumed to reflect processes such as attention switching upon presentation of the task stimulus. However, several acupuncture fMRI studies have interpreted acupuncture-related deactivation patterns as important manifestations of a central modulatory mechanism (Hui et al. 2000; Fang et al. 2012; Hui et al. 2010a, b; Fang et al. 2009; Hui et al. 2005). These studies suggested that regions of deactivation related to acupuncture, mainly located in limbic and paralimbic regions, and represented therapeutic inhibitory effects. It is important to note that there is significant overlap between limbic and paralimbic regions and the DMN; additionally, the only test-retest study conducted on acupuncture-related changes in brain activation to date demonstrated that the reliability of deactivated patterns was much lower than that of activated patterns (Kong et al. 2007b). Accordingly, the specificity and reliability of regional deactivation patterns induced by acupuncture remains controversial and requires verification before it can be interpreted with respect to the potential therapeutic mechanisms of acupuncture.

1.8 Summary

This chapter introduced a number of early studies that used fMRI to investigate the therapeutic effects and mechanisms of acupuncture stimulation. These early studies mainly focused on the characteristics of acupoint specificity, acupuncture sensations, differences among types of acupuncture manipulations, and analgesic mechanism of acupuncture. However, there are many methodological problems with these early studies that call into question the reliability and usefulness of their findings. There is a clear need for more rigorous, high-quality fMRI studies to objectively evaluate the effects and mechanisms associated with acupuncture stimulation.

References

Andrews-Hanna JR, Smallwood J, Spreng RN. The default network and self-generated thought: component processes, dynamic control, and clinical relevance. Ann N Y Acad Sci. 2014;1316:29–52.

Asghar AU, Green G, Lythgoe MF, et al. Acupuncture needling sensation: the neural correlates of deqi using fMRI. Brain Res. 2010;1315:111–8.

Atlas LY, Wager TD. How expectations shape pain. Neurosci Lett. 2012;520(2):140–8.

Bai L, Yan H, Li L, et al. Neural specificity of acupuncture stimulation at pericardium 6: evidence from an FMRI study. J Magn Reson Imaging. 2010;31(1):71–7.

Baxter GD, Bleakley C, McDonough S. Clinical effectiveness of laser acupuncture: a systematic review. J Acupunct Meridian Stud. 2008;1(2):65–82.

Behbehani MM. Functional characteristics of the midbrain periaqueductal gray. Prog Neurobiol. 1995;46(6):575–605.

Beissner F. Functional magnetic resonance imaging studies of acupuncture mechanisms: a critique. Focus Altern Complement Ther. 2011;16(1):3–11.

Beissner F, Henke C. Methodological problems in FMRI studies on acupuncture: a critical review with special emphasis on visual and auditory cortex activations. Evid Based Complement Alternat Med. 2011;2011:607637.

Beissner F, Deichmann R, Henke C, et al. Acupuncture–deep pain with an autonomic dimension? NeuroImage. 2012;60(1):653–60.

Bennett CM, Wolford GL, Miller MB. The principled control of false positives in neuroimaging. Soc Cogn Affect Neurosci. 2009;4(4):417–22.

Berman BM, Lao L, Langenberg P, et al. Effectiveness of acupuncture as adjunctive therapy in osteoarthritis of the knee: a randomized, controlled trial. Ann Intern Med. 2004;141(12):901–10.

Brinkhaus B, Ortiz M, Witt CM, et al. Acupuncture in patients with seasonal allergic rhinitis: a randomized trial. Ann Intern Med. 2013;158:225–34.

Chen SJ, Meng L, Yan H, et al. Functional organization of complex brain networks modulated by acupuncture at different acupoints belonging to the same anatomic segment. Chin Med J. 2012;125(15):2694–700.

Chen JE, Glover GH. Functional magnetic resonance imaging methods. Neuropsychol Rev. 2015;25(3):289–313.

Cho ZH, Chung SC, Jones JP, et al. New findings of the correlation between acupoints and corresponding brain cortices using functional MRI. Proc Natl Acad Sci USA. 1998;95(5):2670–3.

Cho ZH, Chung SC, Lee HJ, et al. Retraction. New findings of the correlation between acupoints and corresponding brain cortices using functional MRI. Proc Natl Acad Sci USA. 2006;103(27):10527.

Cho SY, Jahng GH, Park SU, et al. fMRI study of effect on brain activity according to stimulation method at LI11, ST36: painful pressure and acupuncture stimulation of same acupoints. J Altern Complement Med. 2010;16(4):489–95.

Claunch JD, Chan ST, Nixon EE, et al. Commonality and specificity of acupuncture action at three acupoints as evidenced by FMRI. Am J Chin Med. 2012;40(4):695–712.

Dawidson I, Blom M, Lundeberg T, et al. The influence of acupuncture on salivary flow rates in healthy subjects. J Oral Rehabil. 1997;24(3):204–8.

Deng G, Hou BL, Holodny AI, et al. Functional magnetic resonance imaging (fMRI) changes and saliva production associated with acupuncture at LI-2 acupuncture point: a randomized controlled study. BMC Complement Altern Med. 2008;8:37.

Dhond RP, Yeh C, Park K, et al. Acupuncture modulates resting state connectivity in default and sensorimotor brain networks. Pain. 2008;136(3):407–18.

Eklund A, Nichols TE, Knutsson H. Cluster failure: why fMRI inferences for spatial extent have inflated false-positive rates. Proc Natl Acad Sci USA. 2016;113(28):7900–5.

Elsenbruch S. How positive and negative expectations shape the experience of visceral pain. Handb Exp Pharmacol. 2014;225:97–119.

Fang SH, Zhang SZ, Liu H. Study on brain response to acupuncture by functional magnetic resonance imaging—observation on 14 healthy subjects. Zhongguo Zhong Xi Yi Jie He Za Zhi. 2006;26(11):965–8.

Fang J, Jin Z, Wang Y, et al. The salient characteristics of the central effects of acupuncture needling: limbic-paralimbic-neocortical network modulation. Hum Brain Mapp. 2009;30(4):1196–206.

Fang J, Wang X, Liu H, et al. The limbic-prefrontal network modulated by Electroacupuncture at CV4 and CV12. Evid Based Complement Alternat Med. 2012;2012:515893.

Gareus IK, Lacour M, Schulte AC, et al. Is there a BOLD response of the visual cortex on stimulation of the vision-related acupoint GB 37? J Magn Reson Imaging. 2002;15(3):227–32.

Han JS. Acupuncture analgesia: areas of consensus and controversy. Pain. 2011;152(3 Suppl):S41–8.

He T, Zhu W, SQ D, et al. Neural mechanisms of acupuncture as revealed by fMRI studies. Auton Neurosci. 2015;190:1–9.

Huang ST, Chen GY, Lo HM, et al. Increase in the vagal modulation by acupuncture at neiguan point in the healthy subjects. Am J Chin Med. 2005;33:157–64.

Huang W, Pach D, Napadow V, et al. Characterizing acupuncture stimuli using brain imaging with FMRI—a systematic review and meta-analysis of the literature. PLoS One. 2012;7(4):e32960.

Hui KK, Liu J, Makris N, et al. Acupuncture modulates the limbic system and subcortical gray structures of the human brain: evidence from fMRI studies in normal subjects. Hum Brain Mapp. 2000;9(1):13–25.

Hui KK, Liu J, Marina O, et al. The integrated response of the human cerebro-cerebellar and limbic systems to acupuncture stimulation at ST 36 as evidenced by fMRI. NeuroImage. 2005;27(3):479–96.

Hui KK, Nixon EE, Vangel MG, et al. Characterization of the "deqi" response in acupuncture. BMC Complement Altern Med. 2007;7:33.

Hui KK, Marina O, Claunch JD, et al. Acupuncture mobilizes the brain's default mode and its anti-correlated network in healthy subjects. Brain Res. 2009;1287:84–103.

Hui KK, Marina O, Liu J, et al. Acupuncture, the limbic system, and the anticorrelated networks of the brain. Auton Neurosci. 2010a;157(1–2):81–90.

Hui KK, Napadow V, Liu J, et al. Monitoring acupuncture effects on human brain by FMRI. J Vis Exp. 2010b;38:1190.

Hui KK, Sporko TN, Vangel MG, et al. Perception of Deqi by Chinese and American acupuncturists: a pilot survey. Chin Med. 2011;6(1):2.

Jeun SS, Kim JS, Kim BS, et al. Acupuncture stimulation for motor cortex activities: a 3T fMRI study. Am J Chin Med. 2005;33(4):573–8.

Jiang Y, Wang H, Liu Z, et al. Manipulation of and sustained effects on the human brain induced by different modalities of acupuncture: an fMRI study. PLoS One. 2013;8(6):e66815.

Jiang Y, Liu J, Liu J, et al. Cerebral blood flow-based evidence for mechanisms of low- versus high-frequency transcutaneous electric acupoint stimulation analgesia: a perfusion fMRI study in humans. Neuroscience. 2014;268:180–93.

Jin LM, Qin CJ, Lan L, et al. Local anesthesia at ST36 to reveal responding Brain areas to deqi. Evid Based Complement Alternat Med. 2014;2014:987365.

Kong J, Ma L, Gollub RL, et al. A pilot study of functional magnetic resonance imaging of the brain during manual and electroacupuncture stimulation of acupuncture point (LI-4 Hegu) in

normal subjects reveals differential brain activation between methods. J Altern Complement Med. 2002;8(4):411–9.
Kong J, Gollub R, Huang T, et al. Acupuncture deqi, from qualitative history to quantitative measurement. J Altern Complement Med. 2007a;13(10):1059–70.
Kong J, Gollub RL, Webb JM, et al. Test-retest study of fMRI signal change evoked by electroacupuncture stimulation. NeuroImage. 2007b;34(3):1171–81.
Kong J, Kaptchuk TJ, Polich G, et al. An fMRI study on the interaction and dissociation between expectation of pain relief and acupuncture treatment. NeuroImage. 2009a;47(3):1066–76.
Kong J, Kaptchuk TJ, Polich G, et al. Expectancy and treatment interactions: a dissociation between acupuncture analgesia and expectancy evoked placebo analgesia. NeuroImage. 2009b;45(3):940–9.
Kucyi A, Davis KD. The dynamic pain connectome. Trends Neurosci. 2015;38(2):86–95.
Leung L. Neurophysiological basis of acupuncture-induced analgesia—an updated review. J Acupunct Meridian Stud. 2012;5(6):261–70.
Li G, Liu HL, Cheung RT, et al. An fMRI study comparing brain activation between word generation and electrical stimulation of language-implicated acupoints. Hum Brain Mapp. 2003a;18(3):233–8.
Li G, Cheung RT, Ma QY, et al. Visual cortical activations on fMRI upon stimulation of the vision-implicated acupoints. Neuroreport. 2003b;14(5):669–73.
Li K, Shan B, Xu J, et al. Changes in FMRI in the human brain related to different durations of manual acupuncture needling. J Altern Complement Med. 2006;12(7):615–23.
Li L, Liu H, Li YZ, et al. The human brain response to acupuncture on same-meridian acupoints: evidence from an fMRI study. J Altern Complement Med. 2008;14(6):673–8.
Lin JG, Chen WL. Review: acupuncture analgesia in clinical trials. Am J Chin Med. 2009;37(1):1–18.
Linnman C, Moulton EA, Barmettler G, et al. Neuroimaging of the periaqueductal gray: state of the field. NeuroImage. 2012;60(1):505–22.
Liu WC, Feldman SC, Cook DB, et al. fMRI study of acupuncture-induced periaqueductal gray activity in humans. Neuroreport. 2004;15(12):1937–40.
Liu P, Zhang Y, Zhou G, et al. Partial correlation investigation on the default mode network involved in acupuncture: an fMRI study. Neurosci Lett. 2009;462(3):183–7.
Liu H, JY X, Li L, et al. FMRI evidence of acupoints specificity in two adjacent acupoints. Evid Based Complement Alternat Med. 2013;2013:932581.
MacPherson H, Green G, Nevado A, et al. Brain imaging of acupuncture: comparing superficial with deep needling. Neurosci Lett. 2008;434(1):144–9.
Matthews PM, Jezzard P. Functional magnetic resonance imaging. J Neurol Neurosurg Psychiatry. 2004;75(1):6–12.
Morganstein WM. Acupuncture in the treatment of xerostomia: clinical report. Gen Dent. 2005;53(3):223–7.
Napadow V, Dhond RP, Purdon P, et al. Correlating acupuncture FMRI in the human brainstem with heart rate variability. Conf Proc IEEE Eng Med Biol Soc. 2005a;5:4496–9.
Napadow V, Makris N, Liu J, et al. Effects of electroacupuncture versus manual acupuncture on the human brain as measured by fMRI. Hum Brain Mapp. 2005b;24(3):193–205.
Napadow V, Dhond RP, Kim J, et al. Brain encoding of acupuncture sensation—coupling on-line rating with fMRI. NeuroImage. 2009a;47(3):1055–65.
Napadow V, Dhond R, Park K, et al. Time-variant fMRI activity in the brainstem and higher structures in response to acupuncture. NeuroImage. 2009b;47(1):289–301.
NIH Consensus Conference. NIH consensus conference. Acupuncture. JAMA. 1998;280(17):1518–24.
Poldrack RA. The future of fMRI in cognitive neuroscience. NeuroImage. 2012;62(2):1216–20.
Quah-Smith I, Williams MA, al LT. Differential brain effects of laser and needle acupuncture at LR8 using functional MRI. Acupunct Med. 2013;31(3):282–9.
Raichle ME. The brain's default mode network. Annu Rev Neurosci. 2015;38:433–47.

Scheffold BE, Hsieh CL, Litscher G. Neuroimaging and neuromonitoring effects of electro and manual acupuncture on the central nervous system: a literature review and analysis. Evid Based Complement Alternat Med. 2015;2015:641742.

Seiji O, Yul-Wan S. Functional magnetic resonance imaging. Scholarpedia. 2007;2(10):3105.

Siedentopf CM, Golaszewski SM, Mottaghy FM, et al. Functional magnetic resonance imaging detects activation of the visual association cortex during laser acupuncture of the foot in humans. Neurosci Lett. 2002;327(1):53–6.

Sun J, Qin W, Jin L, et al. Impact of global normalization in FMRI acupuncture studies. Evid Based Complement Alternat Med. 2012a;2012:467061.

Sun J, Zhu Y, Jin L, et al. Partly separated activations in the spatial distribution between de-qi and sharp pain during acupuncture stimulation: an fMRI-based study. Evid Based Complement Alternat Med. 2012b;2012:934085.

Sun J, Zhu Y, Yang Y, et al. What is the de-qi-related pattern of BOLD responses? a review of acupuncture studies in fMRI. Evid Based Complement Alternat Med. 2013;2013:297839.

Wang W, Liu L, Zhi X, et al. Study on the regulatory effect of electro-acupuncture on hegu point (LI4) in cerebral response with functional magnetic resonance imaging. Chin J Integr Med. 2007;13(1):10–6.

Witt C, Brinkhaus B, Jena S, et al. Acupuncture in patients with osteoarthritis of the knee: a randomised trial. Lancet. 2005;366(9480):136–43.

WHO. WHO traditional medicine strategy: 2014–2023. Geneva: World Health Organization; 2014.

Wu MT, Hsieh JC, Xiong J, et al. Central nervous pathway for acupuncture stimulation: localization of processing with functional MR imaging of the brain—preliminary experience. Radiology. 1999;212(1):133–41.

Wu MT, Sheen JM, Chuang KH, et al. Neuronal specificity of acupuncture response: a fMRI study with electroacupuncture. NeuroImage. 2002;16(4):1028–37.

Xiong J, Liu F, Zhang MM, et al. De-qi, not psychological factors, determines the therapeutic efficacy of acupuncture treatment for primary dysmenorrhea. Chin J Integr Med. 2012;18(1):7–15.

Xu SB, Huang B, Zhang CY, et al. Effectiveness of strengthened stimulation during acupuncture for the treatment of Bell palsy: a randomized controlled trial. CMAJ. 2013;185(6):473–9.

Yassa MA. Functional MRI user's guide. 2005. http://pni.med.jhu.edu/intranet/fmriguide/.

Yeo S, Choe IH, van den Noort M, et al. Consecutive acupuncture stimulations lead to significantly decreased neural responses. J Altern Complement Med. 2010;16(4):481–7.

Yin CS, Park HJ, Kim SY, et al. Electroencephalogram changes according to the subjective acupuncture sensation. Neurol Res. 2010;32(Suppl 1):31–6.

Yoo SS, Teh EK, Blinder RA, et al. Modulation of cerebellar activities by acupuncture stimulation: evidence from fMRI study. NeuroImage. 2004;22(2):932–40.

Zhang D, Sun JL, Pieper K. Bivariate mixed effects analysis of clustered data with large cluster sizes. Stat Biosci. 2016;8:220–33.

Zhang WT, Jin Z, Cui GH, et al. Relations between brain network activation and analgesic effect induced by low vs. high frequency electrical acupoint stimulation in different subjects: a functional magnetic resonance imaging study. Brain Res. 2003;982(2):168–78.

Zhong ZP, Wu SS, Liu B, et al. Acupuncture at the acupoints of different meridians at the same anatomy level: a study with functional magnetic resonance imaging. Nan Fang Yi Ke Da Xue Xue Bao. 2010;30(6):1363–5, 1372.

Zyloney CE, Jensen K, Polich G, et al. Imaging the functional connectivity of the periaqueductal gray during genuine and sham electroacupuncture treatment. Mol Pain. 2010;6:80.

Temporospatial Encoding of Acupuncture Effects in the Brain

2

Lijun Bai and Jie Tian

2.1 Introduction

Acupuncture is a traditional Chinese healing modality that has existed for more than 2500 years. In recent decades, acupuncture has gained popularity as an alternative and complementary therapeutic intervention in Western medicine (Hui et al. 2000). Acupuncture has been reported to be effective for the treatment of postoperative dental pain, chemotherapy-induced nausea and vomiting, carsickness and seasickness, and pregnancy-related nausea. Other research has demonstrated the promising utility of acupuncture as an adjunct or alternative treatment for drug addiction, stroke rehabilitation, asthma, headache (including tension headache and migraine), and chronic pain. Moreover, the National Institutes of Health (NIH) issued a consensus stating that acupuncture has fewer and less harmful side effects than pharmacological or surgical interventions, making acupuncture an attractive therapy for many indications.

Evidence from animal studies has demonstrated that acupuncture stimulation can facilitate the release of specific neuropeptides in the central nervous system (CNS) and elicit profound physiological and therapeutic effects (Han 2004; Xing et al. 2007). Studies of electroacupuncture (EA) in rats revealed that both low- and high-frequency stimulations could induce analgesia but their effects differ according to the types of endorphins released (Guo et al. 1996). Deep peripheral acupuncture stimulation has also been reported to activate various brain structures, including the limbic, hypothalamic, and brainstem nuclei (Pomeranz 2001).

L. Bai
The Key Laboratory of Biomedical Information Engineering, Ministry of Education, Department of Biomedical Engineering, School of Life Science and Technology, Xi'an Jiaotong University, Xi'an, China

J. Tian (✉)
CAS Key Laboratory of Molecular Imaging, Institute of Automation, Beijing, China
e-mail: jie.tian@ia.ac.cn

© Springer Nature Singapore Pte Ltd. 2018

J. Tian (ed.), *Multi-Modality Neuroimaging Study on Neurobiological Mechanisms of Acupuncture*, DOI 10.1007/978-981-10-4914-9_2

Although animal research clearly supports the role of specific neural pathways in the mechanisms of acupuncture effects, it is difficult to interpret these studies in the context of the more complex human experience, which includes expectation, emotion, and changes in cognition. With recent advancements in the resolution and sensitivity of the neuroimaging technologies such as positron emission tomography (PET), functional magnetic resonance imaging (fMRI), electroencephalography (EEG), and magnetoencephalography (MEG), it has become more feasible to assess and monitor the neurophysiological effects of acupuncture in the human brain. The wide range of physical effects exerted by acupuncture and its purported efficacy for a compendium of clinical pathologies suggest that the brain may be responsible for transmitting the needle stimulation into signals that restore or facilitate homeostatic balance within and across functional physiological systems (Mann 1992; Jeanette et al. 2000; Kaptchuk 2002; White et al. 2007).

With regard to the temporal effects of acupuncture, many studies have demonstrated that acupuncture can induce sustained effects in the brain even after the cessation of therapy (Bai et al. 2009a; Dhond et al. 2008; Price et al. 1984; Qin et al. 2008, 2011). These studies indicate the existence of time-variant features of acupuncture effects in wide brain networks (Bai et al. 2009b, c; Qin et al. 2011).

2.2 Methods of Analysis for Human Acupuncture Neuroimaging Studies

2.2.1 General Linear Model (GLM) Analysis

Voxel-wise application of a GLM is a standard way to analyze BOLD signal changes in response to a stimulus (e.g., acupuncture).

The GLM is a statistical linear model described by the following equation:

$$Y_i = X_i^{'}\beta + \varepsilon_i \tag{2.1}$$

For the analysis of fMRI data, the given data Y_i at time index i is

$$Y_i = x_{i1}\beta_{i1} + \cdots + x_{ik}\beta_{ik} + x_{i,k+1}\beta_{i,k+1} + \cdots + x_{im}\beta_m + \varepsilon_i = x_i^{'}\beta + \varepsilon_i \tag{2.2}$$

where $x_{i1}, \ldots, x_{ik}$ is the combined effect of k for different stimulus types in scan i and is often assumed to be additive but with different coefficients $\beta_{i1}, \ldots, \beta_{ik}$ that vary from voxel to voxel.

The combined fMRI response is modeled linearly as $x_{i1}\beta_{i1} + \cdots + x_{ik}\beta_{ik}$. The extra "responses" $x_{i,k+1}, \ldots, x_{i,m}$ at time i show the considerable drift over time of some voxels in fMRI time series data. Accordingly, $x_{i,k+1}\beta_{i,k+1} + \cdots + x_{im}\beta_m$ describes the drift. ε_i is the random error.

The GLM aims to test whether the dynamic characteristics of neural responses in specific brain regions relate with some known input function (e.g., experimental design convoluted with hemodynamic function). GLM has arguably become the most widely used method for analyzing fMRI data and has proven particularly powerful for the analysis of event-related designs, given that a sequence of sparse events occurring at random intervals affords a relatively specific predicted response, and good fit is often interpreted in terms of signal evoked by a particular psychological event (Worsley and Friston 1995; Wager et al. 2005). However, when the precise timing and duration of psychological events cannot be specified using a priori defined regressors that model predicted responses to psychological events of interest, the GLM becomes impractical (Lindquist et al. 2007).

2.2.2 Independent Component Analysis (ICA)

The ICA transforms multivariate random signal into signal with multiple statistically independent components. ICA models have traditionally been used to perform blind separation, feature extraction, and signal detection, resulting in the development of many batch and adaptive algorithms. The ICA does not require a priori knowledge or specific assumptions about the time courses of processes contributing to the measured signals. In addition, ICA appears to have a broad developing prospect in the analysis of fMRI data from healthy and clinical populations, especially in the context of unpredictable transient patterns of brain activity associated with psychomotor task performance. A schematic diagram of ICA is shown in Fig. 2.1, where X is the result of multisource signals multiplied by mixing matrix A, $X=AS$. We can obtain the solution of mixing matrix B when S and A are unknown, resulting in $Y=BS$ as the optimal approximation of S.

Given the central limit theorem, the sum of independent random variables tends to follow a Gaussian distribution. Accordingly, the sum of independent random variables should be closer to the Gaussian distribution than any one variable involved. As a consequence, the combination yields the maximization of non-Gaussianity, such that the random variables most remarkably deviating from the Gaussian distribution can be regarded as one independent component of X. This method is called the non-Gaussian maximization method. In addition, there are many other methods used to estimate the ICA, such as approaches to estimate the mutual information minimum and maximum based on the information theory. Many ICA algorithms have been derived from this, such as maximizing or minimizing some related cost function, the adaptive algorithm based on a stochastic gradient, the widely used FastICA algorithm, and the Infomax algorithm. Of note, the Infomax algorithm is commonly used in the analysis of the fMRI data and looks for solutions to a mixed matrix in order to effectively separate multiple Gaussian source signals.

McKeown and colleagues first applied the ICA method as an fMRI analysis in 1998 (McKeown et al. 1998). In this study, the authors demonstrated that ICA could be applied to distinguish artifacts, non-task-related signal components, as well as continuous or temporary assignment-related fMRI activations, based on a weak assumption about their spatial distributions and without a priori knowledge about the time source.

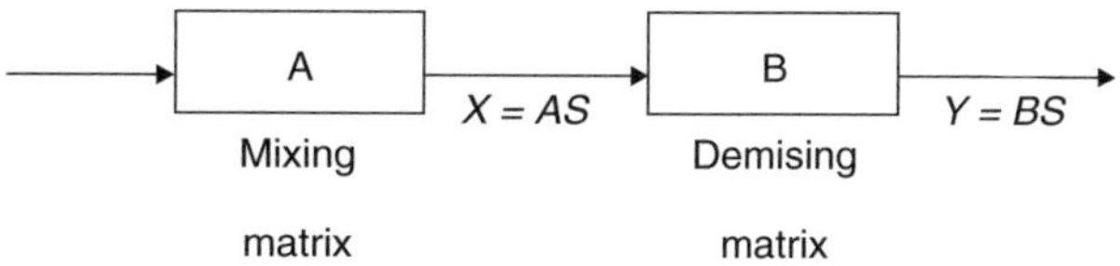

Fig. 2.1 Schematic diagram of the independent component analysis (Reprint with permission from Dai et al. 2013)

The temporal ICA (TICA) algorithm is commonly used under conditions where the times at which signals are collected are mutually independent from one another. In the TICA, data collected from the same voxel in L time points are regarded as a mixed component, so that the whole brain data is composed of M (the number of voxels) mixed components. TICA applied to whole brain data generates a series of independent time series and corresponding brain images.

Spatial ICA (SICA) is commonly used under the assumption that all components are mutually independent from one another, with each source represented as a spatially fixed pattern of activation. In the SICA, voxel-wise data throughout the brain collected at the same time point are regarded as a mixed component, so the whole brain data is composed of L (the number of time points) mixed components. SICA in whole brain data generates a series of independent images and corresponding time series.

2.2.3 Functional Connectivity Analysis

The concept of functional brain connectivity was proposed in early electrophysiological studies. In the early 1990s, Friston et al. introduced the concepts of functional and effective connectivity and applied them to issues in neuroscience (Friston et al. 1993a, b). Functional connectivity was initially defined as a temporal correlation between spatially remote neurophysiological events occurring in a neuroimaging time series. This definition was operational and provided a simple characterization of functional interactions. In 2000, Sporns et al. published a more precise definition of functional connectivity, stating that functional connectivity captures patterns of deviations from statistical independence between distributed and often spatially remote neuronal units, measuring their correlation/covariance, spectral coherence, and phase locking. Of note, functional connectivity does not provide any direct insight into how correlations are mediated (Sporns et al. 2000).

By contrast, effective connectivity can be defined as the influence of one neural system on another, occurring at either a synaptic or cortical level. Some studies have shown that structural equation modeling can be conceived as a linear regression model for effective connectivity, while dynamic causal modeling can improve analyses of brain connectivity to be more akin to analyses of regionally specific effects (Friston 1994; Mclntosh and Gonzalez-Lima 1994; Buchel and Friston 1997; Mechelli et al. 2003).

There are two popular methods for functional connectivity analyses: the seed-based correlation analysis method and the multivariate analysis method, which includes ICA and principal component analysis (PCA) approaches. The specific processing steps for functional connectivity analysis include (1) image preprocessing, including realignment, spatial normalization, spatial smoothing, band-pass filtering, and covariate regression, (2) region-of-interest (ROI) selection to investigate specific regional correlations, (3) calculation of the correlation coefficients between the reference time course (in previous studies, the averaged time courses of voxels within a given ROI) and the BOLD time course from all of other brain voxels, and

(4) normalization of the distribution by applying Fisher's Z transform to the correlation coefficients.

In step 3 of this approach, correlation coefficients less than the given threshold are set to zero. The calculation is described as follows:

$$cc = \frac{\sum_{i=1}^{N}\left(r(i)-\bar{R}\right)\cdot\left(S_i-\bar{S}\right)}{\sqrt{\sum_{i=1}^{N}\left(r(i)-\bar{R}\right)^2\cdot\sum_{i=1}^{N}\left(S_i-\bar{S}\right)^2}} \quad (2.3)$$

where r is the reference time course, S is the signal for a given voxel, $\bar{R}$ is the reference time course for a given voxel, and $\bar{S}$ is the time series for a given voxel. The summation is performed for all time points. Because fMRI time series data can inform both temporal and spatial correlations, it can be expected that the distribution of correlation coefficients will be skewed due to intrinsic temporal and spatial correlations from the imaging method (Friston et al. 1994a; Lowe et al. 1998). The distribution of correlations can differ depending on the ROI selected as the reference for the correlation due to artifacts arising from cardiac, respiratory, or other physiological "noise" during volume collection (Lowe et al. 1998; Hampson et al. 2006).

In step 4, Fisher's Z transform is applied as follows:

$$F = \frac{1}{2}\ln\frac{1+r}{1-r} \quad (2.4)$$

At present, major neuroimaging studies of acupuncture primarily report acupuncture-induced activation patterns. Functional connectivity analyses can be applied to correlations analyses of multi-brain region activation following acupuncture stimulation in order to better inform the neural networks that underlie acupuncture effects.

2.2.4 Time Series State Analysis Algorithm Based on the Change-Point Theory

As mentioned above, although the GLM approach has arguably become the most popular way to analyze fMRI data, it becomes impractical when the precise timing and duration of psychological events cannot be specified a priori. The hierarchical exponentially weighted moving average (HEWMA) model is an approach that allows the predicted signal to depend nonlinearly on the input, using ideas from statistical control theory and change-point theory to model slowly varying processes for which the onset times and durations of underlying psychological activity are uncertain. The HEWMA model is a multi-subject extension of existing EWMA models for individual participants (and accordingly a single time series), adapted to be applicable to a cohort analysis using a hierarchical model. The HEWMA method can thus be used for fMRI data analysis in a voxel-wise manner throughout the

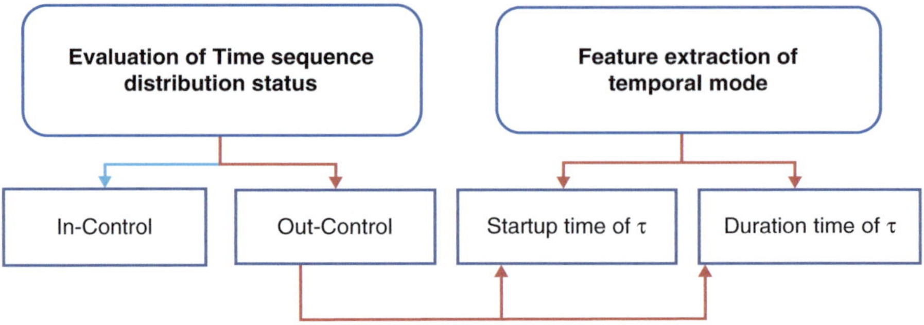

Fig. 2.2 Schematic diagram of the time series state analysis algorithm based on the change-point theory (Reprint with permission from Dai et al. 2013)

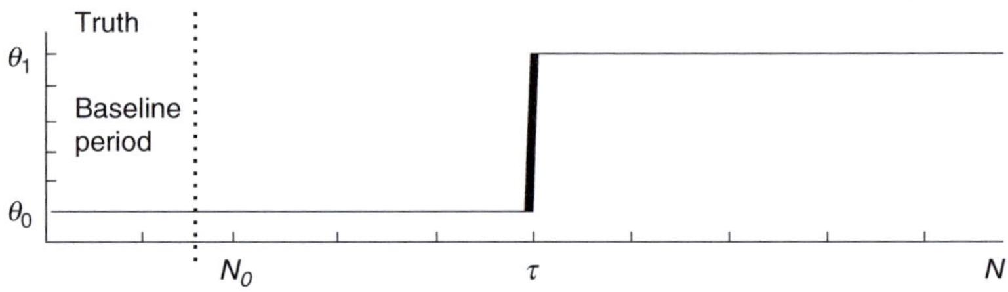

Fig. 2.3 Schematic of the model of true activation (Reprint with permission from Lindquist et al. 2007)

brain, for ROI data, or for temporal components extracted using an ICA or a similar method (Wager et al. 2005; Lindquist et al. 2007).

A schematic diagram of the time series state analysis algorithm based on the change-point theory is shown in Fig. 2.2. Given a process that produces a sequence of observations $\vec{x} = (x_1,,,x_2,,,\ldots,,,x_3)^{\mathrm{T}}$ (e.g., a fMRI time series), a two-state model can be produced where data is modeled as the combination of two normal distributions, one with mean θ_0 and covariance matrix Σ and the other with mean θ_1 and the same covariance. In the baseline acquisition period, the process generates a distribution of data with mean θ_0, and the process in this state is considered to be in control. Observations maintain this distribution until the change point τ, when the process changes (i.e., a new psychological state results in increased or decreased neural activity), generating fMRI observations from the second distribution with mean θ_1 (Fig. 2.3). In this second period, the process is deemed to be out-of-control or in the out-of-control state (Lindquist et al. 2007).

2.3 Acupuncture Neuroimaging Studies in Humans

Noninvasive brain imaging techniques, including positron emission tomography (PET) and fMRI, have provided the opportunity to examine the effects of acupuncture on brain activation. Accordingly, significant modulatory effects of acupuncture have been identified at various levels throughout the CNS. This include the endogenous antinociceptive limbic networks (the cingulate cortex, insula, and hypothalamus) as well as higher-order cognitive and affective control centers within the prefrontal cortex and medial temporal lobe (the amygdala and hippocampus) (Wu et al. 1999, 2002; Hui et al. 2000, 2005; Kong et al. 2002; Zhang et al. 2003; Liu et al. 2004; Yoo et al. 2004; Pariente et al. 2005; Napadow et al. 2007). Here, we will review literature reporting the effects of acupuncture on brain activation.

In 1998, Cho et al. first reported that the vision-related acupoint stimulation at VA1, VA3, and VA8 could activate the primary visual cortex (Cho et al. 1998). However, acupoint specificity has not been fully supported by other fMRI studies. For example, while Cho's results were successfully reproduced by Siedentopf et al. (2002) using laser acupuncture, Gareus et al. (2002) failed to replicate these findings.

Neuroimaging data strongly suggest that acupuncture modulates many distributed cortical and subcortical areas of the brain involved in endogenous antinociception and the pain neuromatrix (Davis et al. 1997; Fields and Basbaum 1999; Hofbauer et al. 2001). Modulation of these areas may contribute to the therapeutic effects of acupuncture by shifting autonomic nervous system (ANS) balance and altering the affective and cognitive dimensions of pain processing (Peets and Pomeranz 1978; Clement et al. 1980). Wu et al. found that stimulation at ST36 produced specific increases in signal intensity of the hypothalamus and nucleus accumbens and specific decreases in signal intensity of the rostral anterior cingulate cortex (ACC), amygdala, and hippocampus (Wu et al. 1999). This evidence supported the hypothesis that acupuncture activates structures of the descending antinociceptive pathway and deactivates multiple limbic areas subserving the affective dimension of pain. Similarly, Hui et al. reported that needle stimulation at LI4 on either the right or left side produced consistent modulation of multiple cortical and subcortical limbic and paralimbic structures; moreover, this stimulation induced a wider range of negative signal changes in the limbic-cerebellar system such as the nucleus accumbens, amygdala, hippocampus, parahippocampus, hypothalamus, anterior cingulate gyrus (BA 24), temporal pole, ventral tegmental area, caudate, putamen, and insula (Fig. 2.4) (Hui et al. 2005). In addition, decreased neural responses were only identified in subjects that experienced deqi sensations not in the subjects who experienced pain sensations during needle manipulation. In contrast, two subjects who experienced sharp pain showed predominately increased signal intensity in the parahippocampus, ACC, posterior cingulate cortex (PCC), and putamen. Given that deqi is thought to play a pivotal role in the therapeutic effect of acupuncture (Takeda and Wessel 1994; Witt et al. 2005), observed decreases in activity in the limbic-cerebellar network may be a central characteristic of acupuncture's therapeutic effect.

Biella et al. (2001) demonstrated that true acupuncture at Zusanli (ST36) and Qi-ze (Lu 5) statistically increased regional cerebral blood flow (rCBF) in the ACC, bilateral insula, bilateral cerebellum, right superior frontal gyrus, and right medial frontal gyrus, whereas sham acupuncture (superficial needle insertion 1 cm lateral to each acupoint) increased rCBF in the raphe nuclei, hypothalamus, and left

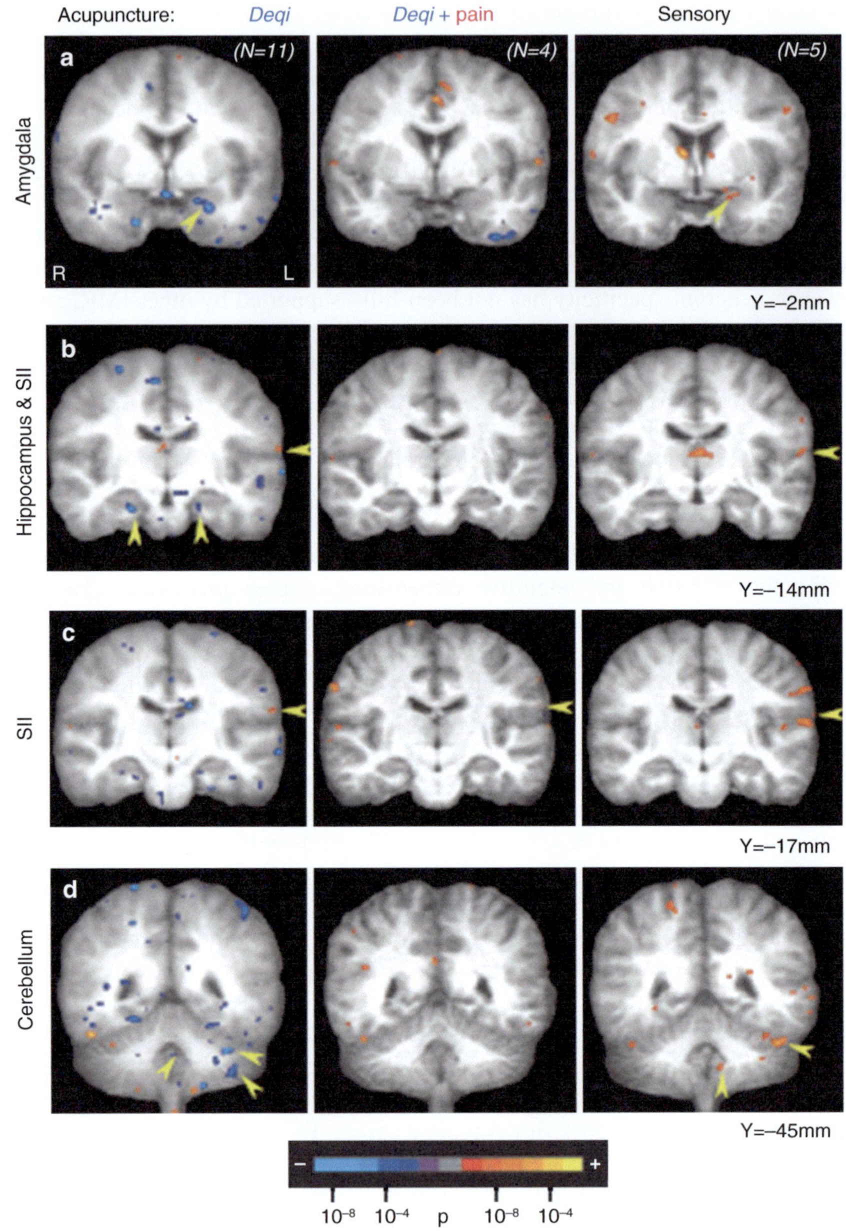

Fig. 2.4 The influence of subjective sensations on fMRI signal changes on major limbic structures, the secondary somatosensory cortex (SII) and the cerebellum during acupuncture at ST36 (Reprint with permission from Hui et al. 2005). (Row **A**) The amygdala showed signal decrease with acupuncture deqi, increase with sensory stimulation, and no significant change with acupuncture mixed sensations. (Row **B**) The hippocampus, bottom arrows, showed signal decrease with acupuncture deqi and no significant change otherwise. (Row **C**) SII, also shown by the right arrows in Row **B**, shows signal increase under all three stimulations. Acupuncture, being a form of sensory stimulation, would be expected to result in signal increases in SII, which is in stark contrast to the widespread signal decreases during acupuncture deqi. (Row **D**) With acupuncture deqi, the cerebellum showed signal decreases in the vermis and lobules VI and VII

temporoparietal junction. Common areas of activation included the claustrum, caudate, putamen, medial and bilateral inferior frontal gyri, and (to a lesser degree) the right anterior insula. Chronic and acute pain can induce activation in pain-related areas including the ACC, insula, and cerebellum. Moreover, the ACC is thought to be involved in the estimation and modulation of sensory and cognitive signals. This is in agreement with indications that the ACC is involved in a number of pain responses, pain anticipatory mechanisms, and pain-related cognitive procedures (Derbyshire et al. 1997; Rainville et al. 1997, 1999; Casey 1999) including attention to pain sensation (Davis et al. 1997).

Yoo et al. reported that acupuncture at PC6 induced the activation of spatially distinct neural substrates, including cerebral structures and areas of the cerebellum such as the declive, nodulus, uvula, quadrangular/superior semilunar lobules, and left cerebellar tonsil. However, neither sham acupuncture nor tactile stimulation elicited cerebellar activation, as shown in Fig. 2.5 (Kong et al. 2002). Liu et al. demonstrated that acupuncture at LI4 (Hegu) but not at a sham acupoint induced activation of the periaqueductal gray (PAG) and moreover reported that

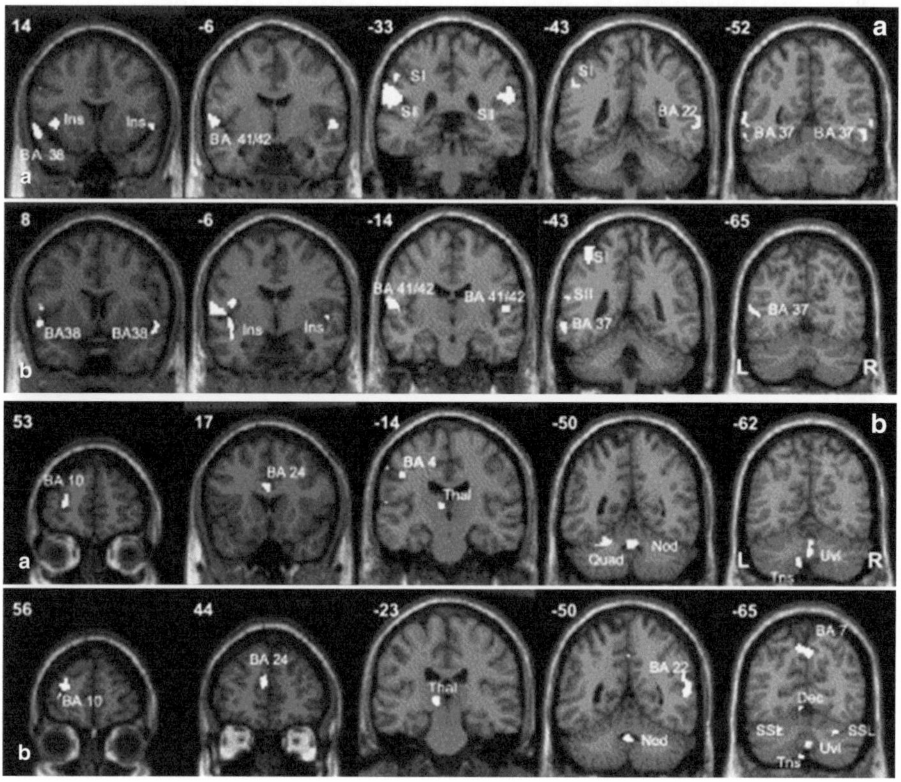

Fig. 2.5 Group activation results among the three different stimulation conditions (Reprint with permission from Yoo et al. 2004). (**a**) Results comparing the rest condition to sham acupuncture and tactile stimulation. Group activation maps are shown for the (A) sham acupuncture > rest condition and (B) tactile stimulation > rest condition. (**b**) Results comparing real acupuncture to sham acupuncture and tactile stimulation. Group activation maps are shown for the (A) real acupuncture > sham acupuncture condition and (B) real acupuncture > tactile stimulation condition

the somatosensory cortex (BA 3, 40) and PAG show distinct activity patterns in response to acupuncture (Liu et al. 2004). Yan et al. found that acupuncture at Liv3 (Taichong) and LI4 (Hegu) but not at sham acupoints activated areas in the middle temporal gyrus and cerebellum and deactivated areas in the middle frontal gyrus and inferior parietal lobule, with some degrees of acupoint specificity. That may reveal that acupuncture at acupoints induces specific patterns of brain activity and these patterns may relate to the therapeutic effects of acupuncture (Yan et al. 2005).

Some studies have demonstrated that different acupuncture manipulations result in different patterns of brain activation. Napadow et al. (2005) reported that EA (particularly at low frequency) produced more widespread fMRI signal increases than manual acupuncture and that all acupuncture stimulations produced more widespread responses than placebo tactile control stimulation. Furthermore, only EA generated significant activation in the anterior middle cingulate cortex (MCC) and pontine raphe area.

2.3.1 Sustained Effects of Acupuncture and Its Influence on fMRI

To date, most neuroimaging studies of acupuncture have mainly focused on the acute impacts of acupuncture on brain activity, adopting the general linear model (GLM) for data analysis. Moreover, a large proportion of previous fMRI studies have employed a block experimental design, which is based on a stimulation-response model in which BOLD signal is assumed to change in response to stimulation and immediately return to the pre-stimulus state after the cessation of stimulation. With this approach, a specific stimulus sequence (i.e., design matrix) is used to define an ideal hemodynamic response function (HRF), which is convolved with the actual hemodynamic response and produces predictors of the BOLD response (Worsley and Friston 1995). Block design fMRI paradigms are useful for detecting activation in response to typical visual or motor tasks, as temporal changes in the BOLD signal conform to the stimulation-response model in these settings. However, a block design may be not valid in cases when a stimulus-response behavior has not been confirmed, as in the case of acupuncture stimulation.

Acupuncture has been shown to exert sustained effects on brain activity even after the cessation of needle stimulation (Price et al. 1984), suggesting that acupuncture effects may have time-variant properties that are acupoint specific. To this end, many clinical reports have indicated that acupuncture produces therapeutic effects that long outlast the duration of actual therapy (Beijing and Nanjing Colleges of Traditional Chinese Medicine 1980). A psychophysical analysis by Price et al. (1984) also suggested that the analgesic effects of acupuncture peak long after the completion of a needling session. On the hypothesis that acupuncture has sustained effects, the temporal aspects of BOLD responses to acupuncture are likely to violate the assumptions of block design GLM estimates (Fig. 2.6) (Bai et al. 2009b) in that

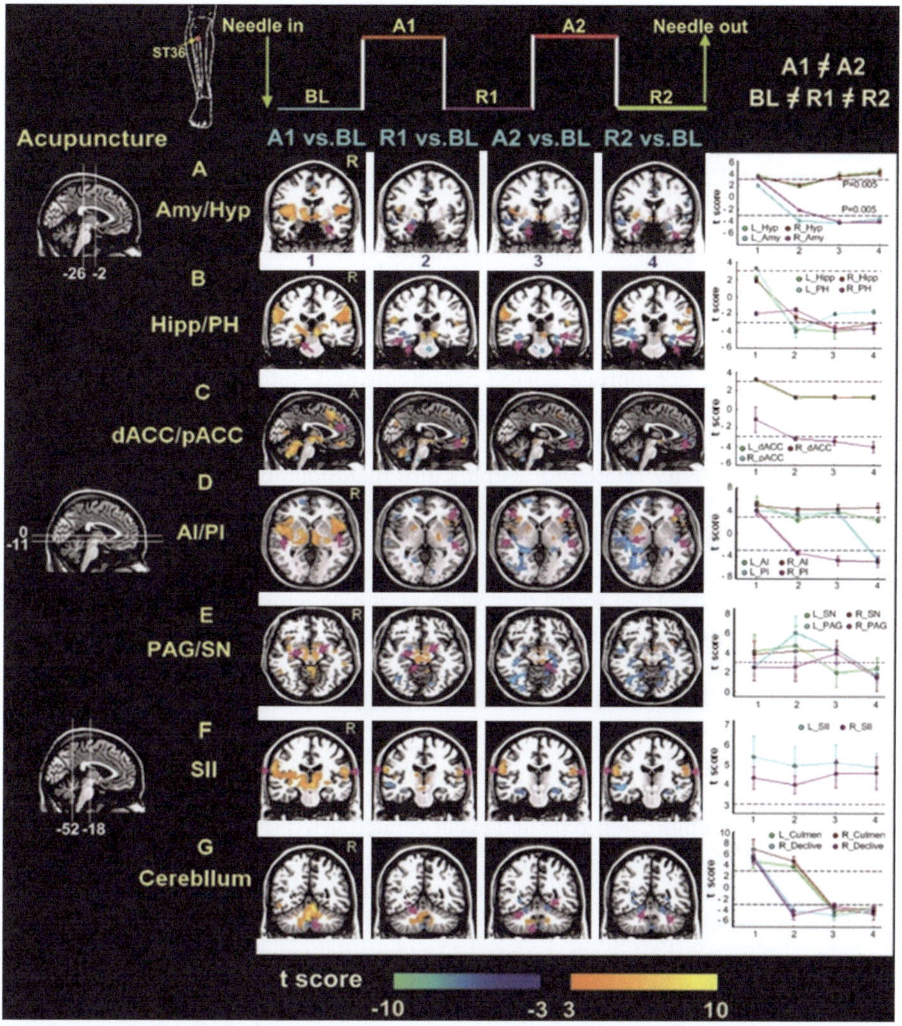

Fig. 2.6 Activity patterns of representative areas in different epochs of multi-block following acupuncture stimulation at ST36 (Reprint with permission from Bai et al. 2009b). Corresponding *t*-values of representative regions in different periods are also indicated. Error bars indicate the standard error of the mean. (**A**, **B**) The amygdala (Amy), hippocampus (Hipp), and parahippocampus (PH) exhibited weakly positive responses in the first stimulation (A1) that decreased to below baseline level thereafter. (**C**) Early positive and negative signal responses were notable in the dorsal and pregenual anterior cingulate cortex (dACC and pACC), respectively, in sequential conditions. (**D**, **F**) The anterior and posterior insula (AI and PI) and secondary somatosensory cortex (SII) exhibited persistently increased responses during the whole trial. (A, E) Episodic responses were primarily distributed in the hypothalamus (Hyp) and brainstem structures (periaqueductal gray, PAG; substantia nigra, SN). The greatest positive activity emerged in R1 and plateaued in A2 but was nonsignificant. (**G**) Early responses in the cerebellum (culmen and declive) were positive and later became negative

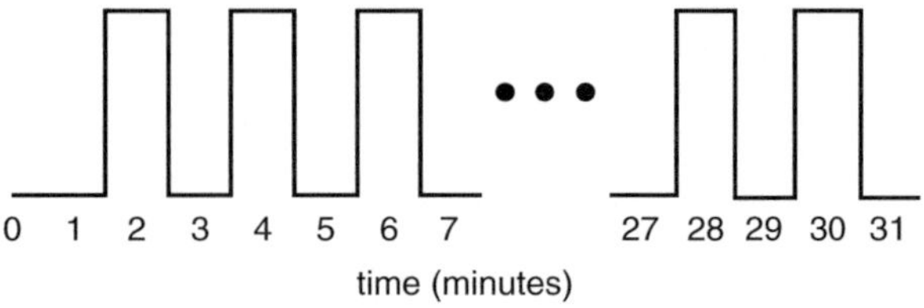

Fig. 2.7 An fMRI block design paradigm consisting of alternating 1-min stimulation (ST36 or sham acupoint) and rest blocks (Reprint with permission from Napadow et al. 2009b)

relevant BOLD responses are unlikely to return to baseline after initial stimulation. Indeed, an investigation using an ICA provided direct evidence that interleaved resting epochs in the block design paradigm retain acupuncture-related changes (Zhang et al. 2009). On the basis that the temporal profile of acupuncture is slow to develop and resolve, more appropriate design paradigms and statistical models should be selected in future studies in order to elucidate the actual effects of acupuncture.

One major obstacle to the multi-block design is the difficulty of distinguishing between brain activity related to acupuncture manipulation itself (e.g., sensation, attention, and cognition) and activity associated with its sustained effects. Napadow et al. (2009a) adopted a long duration (>30 min) stimulus paradigm and compared ST36 acupuncture with sham point acupuncture to evaluate time-variant brain responses (Fig. 2.7). They found that ST36 verum acupuncture modulated activity in the substantia nigra, nucleus raphe magnus, locus coeruleus, nucleus cuneiformis, periaqueductal gray, and limbic areas, whereas both stimulations produced linear decreases in the time-variant activation of sensorimotor brain regions (i.e., the SII, insula, and premotor cortex). These data indicated that acupuncture produces to both early (immediate) and late (30 min after the start of stimulation) phases of brain activation. To address this possibility, Qin et al. (2008) proposed a novel experimental paradigm, non-repeated event-related fMRI (NRER-fMRI), to explore the prolonged effects of acupuncture on resting-state brain networks. Compared with the acupuncture at a nearby non-acupoint, ST36 acupuncture produced higher-level correlations among amygdala-associated networks; these areas mainly included limbic/paralimbic areas (the ACC and insula) and brainstem structures (the PAG) (Fig. 2.8). Similarly, acupuncture but not sham stimulation produced increased connectivity in the default mode network and sensorimotor network (Dhond et al. 2007), including the medial temporal lobe, PAG, and supplementary motor area (SMA). Connectivity between the hippocampus and DMN was also correlated with parasympathetic output following acupuncture stimulation in the abovementioned study. These data indicated that autonomic modulation might represent an important therapeutic mechanism of acupuncture leading to sustained effects, which is consistent with what is known regarding autonomic efferent nerve activity and the analgesic effects of acupuncture (Haker et al. 2000; Hsu et al. 2007; Sakai et al. 2007). In further support of this hypothesis, Baliki et al. (2008) reported differences in resting-state brain functional connectivity between individuals with chronic pain and healthy control subjects and proposed that differences were related to the cognitive and affective components of chronic pain. Future exploration of the alternating interplay between external acupuncture intervention and the reorganization of

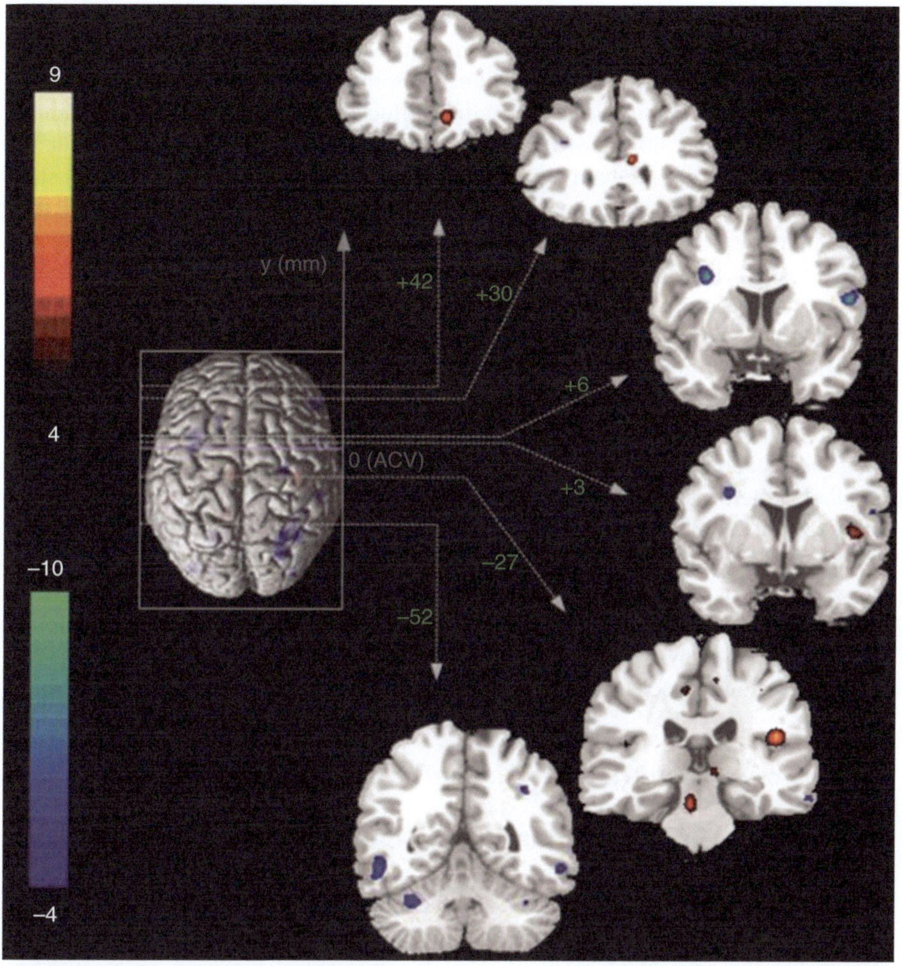

Fig. 2.8 Acupuncture enhanced activity correlations between the amygdala and the insula, anterior cingulate cortex, and periaqueductal gray poststimulus (Reprint with permission from Bai et al. 2009a), whereas sham stimulation enhanced activity correlations between the amygdala and the secondary somatosensory cortex and cerebellum. *ACV*, anterior commissure verticalization

resting-state brain networks in chronic pain patients will better inform our understanding of the mechanism of acupuncture analgesia.

If acupuncture exhibits temporally delayed effects, an understanding of its temporal properties is crucial. One pioneer study developed a novel approach (defining separate models) to evaluate dynamic signal changes between baseline activity and post-acupuncture neural activity in sequential epochs within a multi-block design (Bai et al. 2009b). The results showed that ST36 acupuncture induced time-varied response patterns in limbic-cerebellar and brainstem structures (Fig. 2.6). Moreover, it was noted that some regions only responded to initial acupuncture stimulation (i.e., the PCC), while others exhibited increasing or tapering activities for the duration of the experimental session (i.e., the PAG and rostral ventromedial medulla [RVM]). Further, other brain areas showed sustained responses (i.e., the insula) and continuously exerted controlling and coordinating influences throughout the scan. Limbic and brainstem areas have been indicated to support endogenous antinociceptive mechanisms as part of the pain neuromatrix. In addition, evidence from animal studies suggests that acupuncture analgesia is supported by endogenous opioidergic and/or monoaminergic antinociceptive networks (Hoffman et al. 2005). The PAG and RVM together serve as one such mechanism that modulates ascending nociceptive responses by promoting the release of endogenous opioids (Napadow et al. 2005). The RVM has distinct functional populations of neurons that inhibit (off cells) and facilitate (on cells) nociceptive transmission (Haws et al. 1989; Tortorici and Vanegas 1994). Accordingly, the PAG-RVM network may function as a unit to exerting discrete global control over dorsal horn pain transmission in the context of acupuncture analgesia. In addition, PAG activity is facilitated by top-down processes originating in higher centers such as the insula and ACC (Fields et al. 1991; Urban and Gebhart 1999; Millan 2002; Porreca et al. 2002). These areas, along with limbic regions including the hippocampus and amygdala, comprise the descending antinociceptive pathway. Thus, it can be theorized that the mechanism of acupuncture analgesia may relate to altered pain perception mediated by inhibiting the antinociceptive action in the affective pathway while mobilizing the descending mechanisms by controlling the transmission of nociceptive signals to the brain.

2.4 Brain Network Analysis Methods

2.4.1 Graph Theory in Brain Network Analysis

Brain systems are frequently comprised of smaller, dynamic, and highly interacting subsystems. Graph theory is one method used to study the general features of these systems. In the context of graph theory, dynamic subsystems are represented as network nodes, and subsystem interactions are represented as network edges. Graph theory model differs from traditional network analysis methods in that it is more focused on subsystem interactions than subsystem structure and function.

2.4.1.1 Common Network Parameters According to Graph Theory

The principle of graph theory is summarized in Fig. 2.9. A network consists of two sets: set V of nodes and set E of edges. N, the size of set V, represents the size of the network. Homogeneity among the elements of set V reflects whether nodes in a given network have the same properties. Element $link_{ij}$ in set E is a combination of two elements, node i and node j in set V, and indicates that there is an edge between node i and node j. If (k, j) is an ordered pair, the network can be seen as directed; otherwise, it is undirected. If each element in set E has a different value, the network is a weighted network; otherwise, it is unweighted. Generally, an edge that connects with itself without passing other nodes does not exist in set E, which means that the

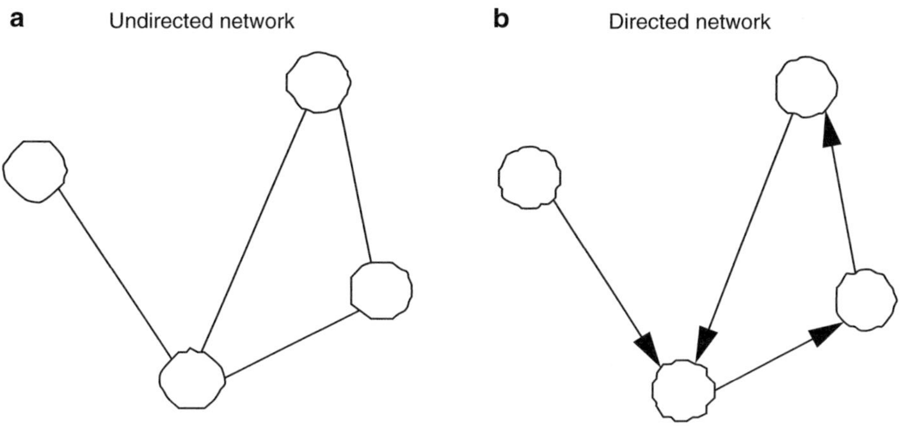

Fig. 2.9 Different kinds of networks according to graph theory (Reprint with permission from Dai et al. 2013). (**a**) Undirected network; (**b**) directed network

combination of *(j, j)* does not exist. Moreover, in an undirected network, there is only one connected edge between two different nodes.

In a network, the path between two nodes is defined as a non-repetitive sequence of nodes and edges passed from one node to another. The length of the path is defined as the sum of the length of mid-edges in the sequence. The shortest length of path is called as characteristic path (*L*). If any two nodes can be reached by a path, the network is a connected network; if a network cannot be connected as a whole, the largest connected network in it is studied and used to make generalizations.

The degree value k_i of any node of a network indicates the sum of nodes that are directly connected with the given node. The degree value can therefore be obtained by summing over the elements of line i in an adjacency matrix; that is to say, $k_i = \sum_j \in v a_j$. If the network is a directed network, the degree of nodes can be divided into two parts, in-degree $ka_i^{in} = \sum a_{ij}$ and out-degree $k_i^{\mathrm{out}} = \sum a_{ij}$, such that the total value of the degree is $k_i = k_i^{\mathrm{in}} + k_i^{\mathrm{out}}$. The degree value accordingly represents the role that a given node plays in a network.

One of the most fundamental properties of a network is degree distribution, which is the probability of randomly selecting a node whose degree value is k. In empirical analysis, the degree distribution is generally represented by the ratio of the number of nodes representing the degree value k to the total number of nodes in a network. Research has shown that the degree distribution of a random network produced by the ER model of Erdos and Renyi follows a Poisson distribution. However, in many complex networks abstracted from real systems (e.g., scientific collaboration networks), degree distributions all follow power law distributions.

Characteristic path length is an important parameter used to describe the inside structure of networks and provides the optimal path for information transfer from one network node to another. This parameter plays a significant role in information transmission and network communication (Pastor-Satorras and Vespignani 2004;

Reijneveld et al. 2007). Moreover, characteristic path length can reflect the efficiency of information transmission of the network on a global scale. The characteristic path length matrix can be used to describe the characteristic path length l_{ij} of any two nodes in a given network, defining the diameter of the network as the longest characteristic path length contained therein. Network mean characteristic path length L describes the average value of the characteristic path length for any two nodes in a given network; that is, $L = 1/N(N-1)\sum_{i}, j \in V, i \neq j l_{ij}$. In general, the characteristic path length matrix is calculated in a connected module. This is because, if a network does not contain unconnected nodes, the characteristic path length of two nodes is infinite. To this end, Newman (2003) developed a method for measuring the mean characteristic path length using the reciprocal of the harmonic average.

The clustering coefficient is another significant parameter to measure the characteristics of a network and is applied to measure the possibility that two nodes adjacent to a third node are also neighbors (Watts 1999). The value of the clustering coefficient C_i of node i equals the ratio of the number of edges (e_i) existing between adjacent nodes to the total possible number of edges among them $k_i(k_i - 1)/2$, which is $C_i = \frac{2e_i}{k_i(k_i-1)} = \frac{\sum_{j,m} a_{ij} a_{jm} a_{mi}}{k_i(k_i-1)}$. The average of the clustering coefficient of all nodes in a given network is the clustering coefficient of the network; that is, $C = \langle C_i \rangle = \frac{1}{N}\sum_{i} \in VC_i$.

A final important network parameter is global efficiency E_{glob}, which can be described as $E_{glob} = 1/N(N-1)\sum_{i}, j \in V, i \in j/l_{ij}$, in which N represents the number of nodes in the network and l_{ij} is the characteristic path length of two nodes in the network. The cost of the network is defined as $k_{cost} = 1/N(N-1)\sum_{i} \in_G k_i$, in which N represents the number of nodes in the network and k_i represents the degree value of node i.

2.4.1.2 The Topological Properties of Small-World Networks and Scale-Free Networks

Complex networks typically fall into two categories: small-world networks (Watts and Strogatz 1998) and scale-free networks (Barabasi and Albert 1999). In the real world, most complex networks have both small-world and scale-free properties at the same time.

The small-world network model was first put forth by Watts and Strogatz (1998). The small-world network has a combination of regular and random network properties and was welcomed with much enthusiasm by the scientific community. In a regular network, the characteristic path length between any two nodes will increase if the network size increases, but the clustering coefficient will not decrease at the same time. In contrast, in a completely random network, the characteristic path length between nodes is short, and the network clustering coefficient is also small. Studies on real-world dynamic processing have shown that there are many shortcuts and edges connecting different areas in a given network, which makes it easier and faster to transfer information between two nodes that are far apart. Although the size of a network might be large, the characteristic path length between nodes can be relatively short, such that the mean characteristic path length L of the network can be described as a geometric logarithm that increases with the growth of the network size N; that is, $L \propto \log(N)$. Of note, the clustering coefficient of a regular network is larger than that of a random network.

Social psychologist Stanley Milgram proposed the concept of six degrees of separation in 1967 based on experimental data statistics (Milgram 1967; Travers and Milgram 1969; Korte and Milgram 1970; Dodds et al. 2003). The six degrees of separation theory states that, in a social network, two strangers can build a connection based on a limited number of acquaintances. That is, more than six steps of separation are required to meet a complete stranger. This phenomenon is also called the small-world phenomenon and exists in many networks (Latora and Marchiori 2001, 2003). Watts and Strogatz pioneered the description of small-world network characteristics, pointing out that a small-world network has a small mean characteristic path length and, unlike the corresponding random network, a large clustering coefficient. These characteristics can be expressed as follows: $\gamma = C_{net}/C_{rand} \gg 1, \lambda = L_{net}/L_{rand} \sim 1$, where rand represents a random network and net represents a real network. From this definition, it can be seen that networks with small-world characteristics have efficient partial and global information processing mechanisms (Stanley 1971).

The concept of the scale-free network was initially proposed by Barabasi and Albert (1999). Barabasi and Albert found that the degree values of many networks in the real world follow a power law distribution; examples include Internet networks, scientific collaboration networks, metabolic networks, and telephone networks. In these networks, the average degree cannot act as a characteristic scale of the network. Therefore, these networks are referred to as scale-free. Moreover, the ability of the node degree to follow a power law distribution is a scale-free characteristic. However, of note, many networks in the real world can follow other distributions including the exponential distribution, Gaussian distribution, and combination distributions.

The power function is a curve that slows gradually, permitting the existence of nodes which have larger degrees in the network. These nodes are hub nodes and can significantly influence the characteristics and functions of the network.

2.4.2 The Application of Graph Theory in Neuroscience Studies

The brain is the most perfect dynamic information processing system known to man. A body of previous research has led to the conclusion that the cerebral cortex is comprised of multiple neural clusters that have partial functional specificities. Neural clusters interact dynamically with one other and build different circuits to support a variety of cognitive activities. An important feature of brain network function is the ability to achieve a balance between functional differentiation and integration. While several experiments in neuroanatomy and electrophysiology have produced information about the data of the channel cortex (Hellwig 2000; Kotter

2001), relatively little is known about the global organization and function of complex functional networks in the brain. New computational methods have been innovated for the study of brain connectivity; of these, graph theory analysis is one useful tool for studying brain network organization principles and characteristics from a global angle.

Indeed, the use of graph theory has begun to flourish in the field of neuroscience, but additional high-quality implementations are required. Previous studies have focused on brain activities during cognitive tasks and considered different regions as different nodes in a complex interactive network. In these studies, interrelations and functional correlations among different brain regions serve as network edges.

Watts and Strogatz (1998) used the graph theory method to identify small-world characteristics in the nervous system. A complex network quantitative method was employed in *C. elegans*, where each neuron was regarded as a node and synaptic connections were regarded as edges. This resulted in a directed network consisting of 282 nodes and 2462 edges. Using this model, Watts and Strogatz discovered that the topological structure of the *C. elegans* network was neither random nor regular network but instead had small-world features.

Salvador et al. (2005) was the first to employ graph theory for the analysis of brain fMRI data. The whole human brain was divided into 90 ROIs (45 for each cerebral hemisphere), and correlations between the resting-state BOLD signals of any two regions were calculated to build the functional network. Salvador and colleagues subsequently analyzed the clustering coefficient and mean characteristic path length of the resultant network and confirmed the presence of small-world characteristics in the resting-state human brain. The authors also identified the presence of subnetworks with long-distance functional connectivity using a cluster analysis.

Achard and colleagues studied the properties of brain networks at different frequencies using wavelet transformations (Achard et al. 2006) and found that small-world characteristics were most notable at low frequencies (0.03–0.06 Hz). Moreover, the degree distributions of human brain networks were found to follow a truncated power law distribution. Fair et al. applied graph theory to developmental neuroscience research and found that human brain development reveals the process of network organization (Fair et al. 2007). It was found that the merging and separation of brain network modules occurred simultaneously, decreasing the number of short edges and increasing the number of long edges over the course of development (Fair et al. 2009). The synthesis of the default network was directly observed during development (Fair et al. 2008).

The above studies all regarded information from one brain region as a single network node. Instead, van den Heuvel et al. studied the brain network at a voxel level (van den Heuvel et al. 2008) and found that voxel-level brain networks also exhibit small-world characteristics. Accordingly, it can be interpreted that the characteristics of human brain networks are robust. However, the power law distribution of degree values in voxel-level brain networks was found to diverge from that in brain region-level networks.

In recent years, graph theory has also been applied to study brain network abnormalities in patients. Supekar et al. (2008) discovered that small-world characteristics were diminished in Alzheimer's disease patient brain networks, specifically manifesting as smaller clustering coefficients with respect to healthy brain networks. This variation was proposed as an index for distinguishing patients from healthy individuals. However, in work performed around the same time, He et al. (2008) demonstrated larger clustering coefficients and mean characteristic path lengths in patients relative to healthy individuals.

Liu et al. (2008) used graph theory to study network characteristics in schizophrenic patients and found that both clustering coefficients and network efficiency were decreased, while the characteristic path length was increased in patients relative to healthy control subjects. In attention-deficit/hyperactivity disorder research by Wang et al. (2009), partial increases in network efficiency were noted although global efficiency was unchanged. Most recently, in 2009, Liu and colleagues evaluated brain network characteristics in individuals with heroin addiction (Liu et al. 2009). The results showed that individuals with heroin addiction retained small-world brain network characteristics but the small-world parameter γ was markedly decreased with respect to healthy control subjects.

2.4.3 The Application of Graph Theory in Acupuncture Studies

In recent years, researchers have begun to apply graph theory to the study of acupuncture (Liu et al. 2010; Qin et al. 2011). The results of these studies showed that after acupuncture therapy, brain network connectivity exhibited time-variant alterations, indicating a lasting effect of acupuncture on network reorganization. Differences noted between the brain network connection modes of the acupuncture and control groups indicated that the anterior insula was significantly involved in acupuncture's effect. In future research on the mechanisms of acupuncture, graph theory should be employed to provide further insight into the effects of acupuncture on signal processing efficiency, brain network connectivity, and network structure.

2.4.4 Analytical Algorithms Based on Pattern Classification

A fundamental content of cognitive neuroscience is to determine how information is represented in neural activation patterns. For this purpose, fMRI is an invaluable tool. Tens of thousands of millions of voxels of data can be produced by fMRI within a matter of seconds; however, the large sizes of these datasets and high levels of inherent noise complicate the use of these datasets for informing cognitive processes (Norman et al. 2006). Acupuncture stimulation usually produces the synchronous activation multiple voxels, resulting in temporal patterns on time series. As mentioned earlier in this chapter, the GLM method is a common analysis approach, but this method is not useful for multi-voxel analyses. Therefore, alternative data analysis methods are required to process this type of fMRI data, particularly for the purposes of acupuncture research.

As mentioned in Chap. 1, Hui and colleagues offered the notable hypothesis that acupuncture produces limbic system deactivation and published several high-level academic papers on the subject (Hui et al. 2000; Smith et al. 2005). This hypothesis theorizes that acupuncture can cause widespread signal deactivation, especially in the limbic system-cerebellar neurocyte, as part of a complex multisystem effect. To address this hypothesis, it is necessary to focus on characteristics of the spatial distribution of brain activation mode under the condition of acupuncture stimulation. Multi-voxel pattern analysis (MVPA) provides a solution to achieve this purpose. MVPA is a data-driven analysis method that does not restrict the analysis of fMRI data to the voxel level. Specifically, MVPA attempts to improve the extraction of neural response activation areas by integrating information on a multi-voxel level. Compared with traditional methods for fMRI analysis, MVPA offers several benefits: first, MVPA provides increased sensitivity; second, increased sensitivity afforded by MVPA methods makes it feasible to measure the presence/absence of cognitive states based on only a few seconds' worth of brain activity data. If the cognitive states in question are sufficiently distinct from one another, discrimination can be made with acceptable statistical significance. MVPA methods can also be used to characterize how these cognitive states are represented in the brain (Norman et al. 2006). Machine learning theory supplements MVPA with a variety of classification algorithms, such as neural network, linear discriminant analysis, and support vector machine algorithms. A brief introduction of basic steps involved in the MVPA method is provided in Fig. 2.10 and summarized here.

1. A multi-block experimental design is used for feature selection (Fig. 2.10a). During scanning, the subject receives two types of visual stimulation: in the example, one is a picture of a bottle, while the other is a picture of a shoe. The purpose of this design is to investigate whether it is possible to judge the kind of stimulation that the subject is receiving according to the gray value of voxels in the cerebral cortex on fMRI data. Therefore, to extract special pattern, we need to select a group of voxels. The gray value of a group of voxels is used to build the feature vector of the present brain activation mode. Moreover, the constructed feature vectors are used in the next step of pattern classification in order to allow the classification of brain activation states.
2. Next is integration of the collected fMRI data (Fig. 2.10b); that is, the fMRI time series of the whole brain for every subject is divided and recombined according to stimulation condition. This is the matrix of feature vectors. Inside of feature vectors are the signal values of voxels in the selected voxel group at specific time points. Given that the stimulation conditions correspond with every feature vectors, the characteristic data must next be divided into two sets: a training set and testing set.
3. Next, the training set is used for to train the sorting machine (Fig. 2.10c). Obtaining discriminant forms of classification and entering the new feature vectors, we can estimate the category of each feature vector.

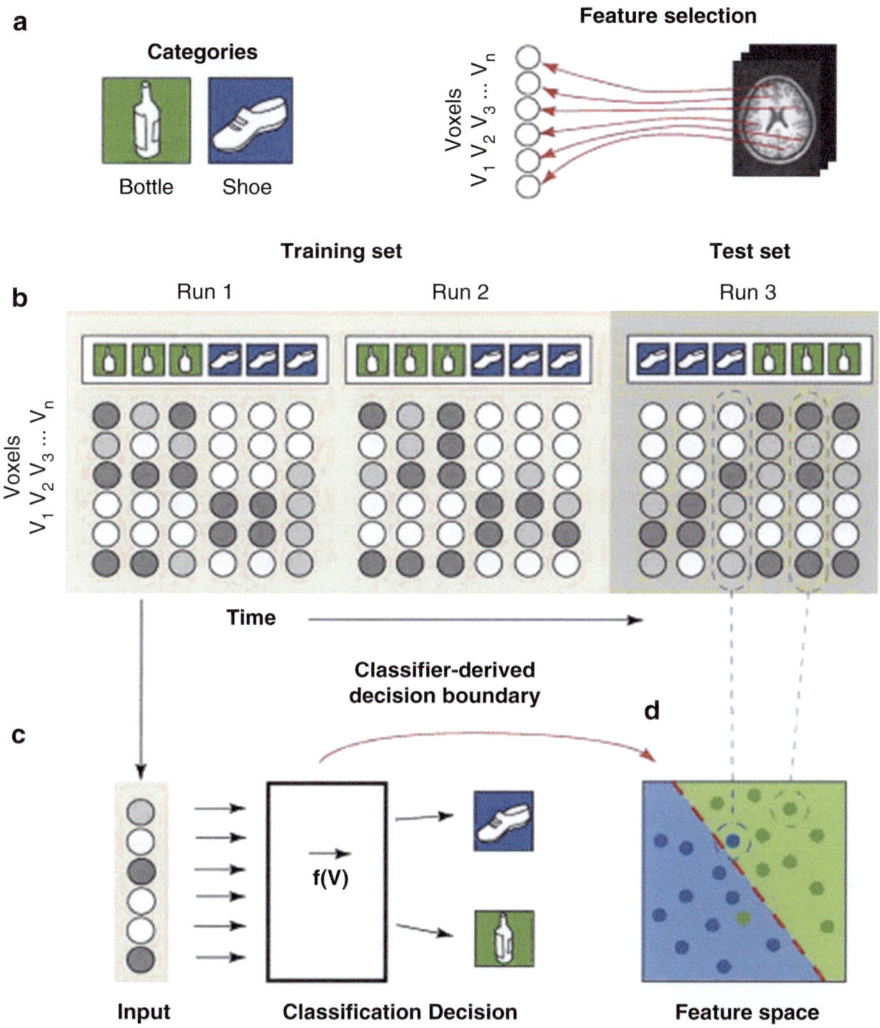

Fig. 2.10 A summary of the multi-voxel pattern analysis method (Reprint with permission from Dai et al. 2013)

4. Next, the trained sorting machine defines a high-dimension voxel model space (compressed into two-dimensional space for the purpose of display; Fig. 2.10d). The red imaginary line is the boundary for classification. Every point in Fig. 2.10d corresponds to a feature vector; that is, a brain activation mode at a specific time point (green and blue correspond to the two stimulation conditions, respectively). The color of the background represents the class of the field to which the feature vector selected by the sorting machine belongs. In the picture, this includes an activation mode that is correctly classified as the bottle picture stimulation (indicated by the green dotted line) and an activation mode classified as the shoe picture stimulation.

Of note, in order to avoid signal deficiencies when applying the MVPA algorithm, smoothing of the voxel signal space should generally be omitted from the fMRI preprocessing protocol; although averaging spaces is an efficient way to decrease noise, it can also obscure meaningful activation signals that can be used to distinguish activation modes, including signal related to the judgment of information and subtle texture patterns of the space mode.

Selection of the sorting machine is another important consideration when applying the MVPA algorithm. As abovementioned, machine learning theory provides a wide variety of classification algorithms for MVPA. The MVPA method commonly adopts a linear discriminant machine (e.g., neural network, linear discriminant analysis, or support vector machine), which calculates the weighted average of voxel gray value, inputs the weighted average as a discriminant equation, and then confirms the category to which the pattern belongs using an effective threshold. Although traditional pattern analysis theory indicates that a nonlinear training machine has a wider range of application than linear training machines, there is no evidence to support this concept in the context of MVPA (Cox and Savoy 2003). Moreover, some research indicates that the results obtained from nonlinear machine methods are more difficult to interpret (Kamitani and Tong 2005). Therefore, a linear support vector machine is recommended for investigating the corresponding neural activation modes stimulated by acupuncture.

According to the MVPA method, characteristics are attributed to large groups of voxels such that even slight responses can lead to the observation of gradual changes under different conditions. Examples of experimental contexts where MVPA has been applied successfully include distinguishing between the visual observation of different object categories, invisible differences between line orientations, and natural scenes. MVPA can also be used to draw conclusions about the neural manifestations underlying a given phenomenon or behavior (Oosterhof et al. 2011). For this purpose, some researchers have combined a ROI-based analysis with the MVPA approach to study characteristics of activation among groups of specific voxels. Although an ROI-based method is appropriate in some cases, the a priori designation of ROI edges is a complex procedure when used in tandem with MVPA. When comparing voxel-based and surface-based methods, it is noteworthy that surface-based methods can provide higher-quality alignment and easier visualization.

The searchlight method is another way in which MVPA can be used to sensitively identify regions encoding specific stimulation types. By moving a searchlight among every voxel, a map of information about the different criteria of interest in the experiment is provided. Conventionally, the searchlight is conceived as a volume sphere that is small enough to have functional anatomical significance with respect to the surface of the cerebral cortex. For information mapping, Oosterhof et al. (2011) performed voxel by utilizing a cortical surface reconstruction. This method diverges from traditional volume-based MVPA in two manners: first, cortical surface reconstruction doesn't utilize voxels that are not a part of the gray matter identified by the anatomical scan. Second, it uses a surface-based geodesic distance metric to define neighborhoods of voxels and does not select voxels across a sulcus.

Additional researches are required to understand how these two differences influence the validity of category creation and the spatial characteristics of the obtained information map. Oosterhof et al. (2011) applied this method to fMRI data obtained while subject to pressed a button with one of their fingers. Surface-based MVPA, especially the information mapping component, was more sensitive than a volume-based approach for measuring information content in this experiment. In addition, surface-based MVPA provided more accurate spatial selectivity.

Currently, the use of fMRI to study acupuncture mainly employs a multi-block experimental design. Similar to the former (Hui et al. 2000; Cox and Savoy 2003; Kong et al. 2009), we can apply multi-block experimental design but applied MVPA at each stimulation or rest condition.

Pattern selection is one of the most important steps for the MVPA method, as the final result largely depends on this process. Therefore, it is necessary to extract the feature vector which best reflects the spatial distribution of the central nervous system activation mode; that is, the gray voxel value vector most likely to be included in activated regions. There are two main method of selecting the feature vector for this purpose:

1. Find out which clusters of the cerebral cortex will be activated under some specific condition based on a priori information (e.g., neuroanatomy or physiology) to determine the ROI. For example, if the experiment only involves visual stimulation, researchers may select a region from occipital lobe to make the feature vector.
2. Base the selection on the statistical result of a traditional general linear model. Application of a traditional general linear model data analysis can yield a statistical parametric map. In this map, every voxel has a corresponding value of t, where t is used to reflect the degree of activation of voxels. Therefore, the t-value can be utilized to make an appropriate threshold; voxels with a t-value higher than the threshold can be put into the voxel group used for extracting the feature vector. For traditional fMRI analysis methods, the statistics of any voxel groups can be used as a basis for selecting the feature vector.

Of note, pattern selection according to a traditional general linear model still has many problems. Although the threshold is quite low during the process of feature vector extraction, if we consider voxels which were not selected as a whole, these regions may contain information relevant to the stimulation-specific activation mode. Therefore, we can use multi-voxel pattern selection method to take the place of the single-mask pattern selection method. Importantly, multi-voxel pattern selection can consider information from whole groups of voxels. Of course, because of the large number of voxels that comprise the entire cerebral cortex, it is computationally difficult to consider all voxels in the brain, even with a multi-voxel pattern selection method. Given that interest is only in specific voxels that can distinguish a given central nervous system activation mode, and considering the functional connections between adjacent voxels, searchlight is an appropriate choice as a pattern selection method (Mitchell et al. 2004).

Comparing the analysis results of MVPA and those obtained from a traditional general linear model, it is clear that MVPA provides a more meaningful basis for determining acupoint specificity. Although the traditional general linear model method has some utility, it lacks sufficient sensitivity and the ability to detect subtle differences in spatial activation patterns. MVPA is a preferable and sufficiently powered method for identifying differences in spatial activation between true and sham conditions in acupuncture studies.

2.5 The Temporospatial Encoding of Acupuncture Effects on Brain Networks

The topological structure of a brain network has a significant effect on its function and dynamic behavior. In neural networks, topological structure refers to the paths for movement of neural information. Anatomical research has verified some fundamental properties of cortical connections; local connections between nerve cells are on the order of a few 100 mm (Le et al. 1991). In addition, long-distance neural connections exist inside the brain, connecting different regions in the cerebral cortex. These long-distance neural connections allow rapid interactions among distant brain regions (Kong et al. 2002). Indeed, these local and long-distance connections provide a good balance between specificity of local brain function and global brain functional integration. However, the experimental quantization and measurement of global properties are still in its early stages of development, and new computing methods for assessing large amounts of information about brain functional connections are a great need. This need is emphasized by a shifting focus of research to functional brain network connectivity (Albert et al. 2000; Achard et al. 2006; Achard and Bullmore 2007; Dhond et al. 2008; Buckner et al. 2009; Bullmore and Sporns 2009; Wang et al. 2010).

Given the complex effects of acupuncture on multiple systems in the human body (Rainville et al. 1997), it is logical that a similar complexity is encountered in the study of acupuncture effects on the brain. In recent years, the "point-to-point" simple research approach of examining simple correlations between spatial activation and acupuncture has proven to be insufficient. Recently, a top acupuncture research group at Massachusetts General Hospital published the first paper about acupoint specificity from a network perspective (Dhond et al. 2008). In this paper, obvious differences in functional brain networks were identified between acupoint and sham (non-acupoint) simulation conditions. In the same year, a preliminary report was published on acupoint specificity and the a priori information network (Qin et al. 2008). In this article, a clear specific effect of Zusanli point acupuncture was demonstrated on amygdala brain networks. These results are perhaps the first to support the theory of acupoint specificity in a scientifically and methodologically robust manner.

In this section, we have considered the effects of acupuncture on the central nervous system as temporally complex with network-level impact and recommended the application of graph theory to describe complex correlations and system-level changes in the brain. By mapping the activities and functional connections of brain regions involved in acupuncture and compiling these interactions into a complete network, we can gain a better understanding of acupuncture and the ways in which it can be used in the clinical context. Further, graph theory analyses offer a unique possibility for novel perspectives on medical diagnosis and treatment. Improved understanding of topological network structure and subsystem organization in the brain will provide a new path for acupuncture research.

2.6 Summary

Acupoint specificity lies at the core of traditional acupuncture theory; the clinical effectiveness of acupuncture is said to depend upon the specific placement of the needles at designated acupuncture points (Kaptchuk 2002). However, neuroimaging evidence supporting the specificity of acupuncture modulatory effects is conflicting. Previous studies have only investigated the spatial distribution of neural responses to acupuncture at specific acupoints, such that temporal information and more complex network-level information have been ignored. As aforementioned, the kinetics of acupuncture is inherently complex and time dependent. An accurate interpretation of acupuncture actions may therefore depend on how effectively we can characterize the nature of temporal variations in brain responses. Moreover, a majority of previous acupuncture neuroimaging research is fraught with methodological challenges, such that these studies may not have sufficiently addressed the complexities of the therapeutic mechanisms of acupuncture. Variability in needling technique, deqi sensations, design paradigm, differences in neuroimaging hardware and software, and data post-processing methods (Smith et al. 2005; Kong et al. 2007) are all likely to account for reported differences in brain responses between studies. Therefore, it is critical to define a standardized system for reporting the details of acupuncture manipulation (MacPherson et al. 2002). In addition, it is necessary to improve and standardize the use of sham or control stimulations in acupuncture studies. A particularly useful approach is the retractable non-penetrating sham needle (Streitberger and Kleinhenz 1998), which gives the impression of skin penetration without piercing the skin and can control for nonspecific cognitive factors known to confound acupuncture studies. Alternatively, sham (nearby non-acupoint) acupuncture can be used to control for physiological responses unrelated to acupoint specificity. Lastly, more appropriate paradigms such as the non-repeated event-related design paradigm should be implemented in future acupuncture studies (Cox and Savoy 2003). An appropriate paradigm in tandem with the implementation of data-driven analysis methods (free of any hypothesis about the temporal profile of acupuncture-related changes) will better inform the effects of acupuncture in the human brain.

This chapter briefly reviewed a variety of literature regarding the neurophysiological mechanisms of acupuncture and modern functional neuroimaging techniques useful for better understanding these mechanisms. Future studies evaluating the central and peripheral effects of needle stimulation in a well-controlled disease model will assist the identification of which neurological substrates contribute to acupuncture's specific clinical effects. Concurrent physiological measurements (e.g., electrocardiography, pupillometry, and electrodermal activity) should also be adopted in conjunction with neuroimaging techniques to help correlate acupuncture-related neural responses with ANS functions. It is our hope that, as advancements in modern neuroimaging facilitate the further exploration of this ancient therapy, horizons will be broadened and the clinical implementation and utility of acupuncture will be enhanced.

References

Achard S, Bullmore E. Efficiency and cost of economical brain functional networks. PLoS Comput Biol. 2007;3(2):e17.

Achard S, Salvador R, Whitcher B, et al. A resilient, low-frequency, small-world human brain functional network with highly connected association cortical hubs. J Neurosci. 2006;26(1):63–72.

Albert R, Jeong H, Barabá si AL. Error and attack tolerance of complex networks. Nature. 2000;406(6794):378–82.

Bai L. The sustained effects of acupuncture. Doctoral dissertation, Xidian University; 2009c.

Bai L, Qin W, Liang J, et al. Spatiotemporal modulation of central neural pathway underlying acupuncture action: a systematic review. Curr Med Imaging Rev. 2009a;5(3):167–73.

Bai L, Qin W, Tian J. Time-varied characteristics of acupuncture effects in fMRI studies. Hum Brain Mapp. 2009b;30(11):3445–60.

Baliki MN, Geha PY, Apkarian AV, et al. Beyond feeling: chronic pain hurts the brain, disrupting the default-mode network dynamics. J Neurosci. 2008;28(6):1398–403.

Barabasi A-L, Albert R. Emergence of scaling in random networks. Science. 1999;286(5439):509–12.

Beijing S, Nanjing Colleges of Traditional Chinese Medicine. Essentials of Chinese acupuncture. Beijing: Foreign Language Press; 1980.

Biella G, Sotgiu ML, Pellegata G, et al. Acupuncture produces central activations in pain regions. NeuroImage. 2001;14:60–6.

Buchel C, Friston KJ. Modulation of connectivity in visual pathways by attention: cortical interactions evaluated with structural equation modeling and fMRI. Cereb Cortex. 1997;7(8):768–78.

Buckner RL, Sepulcre J, Talukdar T, et al. Cortical hubs revealed by intrinsic functional connectivity: mapping, assessment of stability, and relation to Alzheimer's disease. J Neurosci. 2009;29(6):1860–73.

Bullmore E, Sporns O. Complex brain networks: graph theoretical analysis of structural and functional systems. Nat Rev Neurosci. 2009;10(3):186–19.

Casey KL. Forebrain mechanisms of nociception and pain: analysis through imaging. Proc Natl Acad Sci U S A. 1999;96:7668–74.

Cho ZH, Chung SC, Jones JP, et al. New findings of the correlation between acupoints and corresponding brain cortices using functional MRI. Proc Natl Acad Sci U S A. 1998;95(5):2670–3.

Clement JV, McLoughlin L, Tomlin S, et al. Increased beta-endorphin but not met-enkephalin levels in human cerebrospinal fluid after acupuncture for recurrent pain. Lancet. 1980;2(8201):946–9.

Cox DD, Savoy RL. Functional magnetic resonance imaging (fMRI) "brain reading": detecting and classifying distributed patterns of fMRI activity in human visual cortex. NeuroImage. 2003;19(2):261–70.

Dai R, Han J, Shi X, et al. Modern acupunctomics: Zhejiang Science and Technology Publisher; 2013.

Davis KD, Taylor SJ, Crawley AP, et al. Functional MRI of pain- and attention-related activations in the human cingulate cortex. J Neurophysiol. 1997;77:3370–80.

Derbyshire SW, Jones AK, Gyulai F, et al. Pain processing during three levels of noxious stimulation produces differential patterns of central activity. Pain. 1997;73:431–45.

Dhond RP, Witzel T, Yeh C et al. Spatiotemporal mapping the neural correlates of acupuncture. 13th Annual Organization for Human Brain Mapping Conference; 2007; Chicago.

Dhond RP, Yeh C, Park K. Acupuncture modulates resting state connectivity in default and sensorimotor brain networks. Pain. 2008;136:407–18.

Dodds PS, Muhamad R, Watts DJ. An experimental study of search in global social networks. Science. 2003;301(5634):827–9.

Fair DA, Dosenbach NU, Church JA, et al. Development of distinct control networks through segregation and integration. Proc Natl Acad Sci U S A. 2007;104(33):13507–12.

Fair DA, Cohen AL, Dosenbach NU, et al. The maturing architecture of the brain's default network. Proc Natl Acad Sci U S A. 2008;105(10):4028–32.

Fair DA, Cohen AL, Power JD, et al. Functional brain networks develop from a "Local to Distributed" organization. PLoS Comput Biol. 2009;5(5):e1000381.

Fields HL, Basbaum AI. Central nervous system mechanisms of pain modulation. In: Wall PD, Melzack R, editors. Textbook of pain. Edinburgh: Churchill Livingstone; 1999. p. 309–29.

Fields HL, Heinricher MM, Mason P. Neurotransmitters in nociceptive modulatory circuits. Annu Rev Neurosci. 1991;14:219–45.

Friston KJ. Functional and effective connectivity in neuroimaging: a synthesis. Hum Brain Mapp. 1994;2:56–78.

Friston KJ, Frith CD, Fiddle PF, et al. Functional connectivity: the principal component analysis of large (PET) data sets. J Cereb Blood Flow Metab. 1993a;13(1):5–14.

Friston KJ, Frith CD, Frackowiak RS. Time-dependent changes in effective connectivity measured with PET. Hum Brain Mapp. 1993b;1:69–80.

Friston KJ, Jezzard P, Turner R. Analysis of functional MRI time-series. Hum Brain Mapp. 1994a;1:153–71.

Gareus I, Lacour M, Schulte AC, et al. Is there a bold response of the visual cortex on stimulation of the vision-related acupoint GB 37? J Magn Reson Imaging. 2002;15(3):227–32.

Guo HF, Tian J, Wang X, et al. Brain substrates activated by electroacupuncture (ea) of different frequencies (ii): role of fos/jun proteins in EA-induced transcription of preproenkephalin and preprodynorphin genes. Brain Res Mol Brain Res. 1996;43(1–2):167–73.

Haker E, Egekvist H, Bjerring P. Effect of sensory stimulation (acupuncture) on sympathetic and parasympathetic activities in healthy subjects. J Auton Nerv Syst. 2000;79:52–9.

Hampson M, Tokoglu F, Sun Z, et al. Connectivity–behavior analysis reveals that functional connectivity between left BA39 and Broca's area varies with reading ability. NeuroImage. 2006;31:513–9.

Han JS. Acupuncture: neuropeptide release produced by electrical stimulation of different frequencies. Trends Neurosci. 2004;26:17–22.

Haws CM, Williamson AM, Fields HL. Putative nociceptive modulatory neurons in the dorsolateral pontomesencephalic reticular formation. Brain Res. 1989;483:272–82.

He Y, Chen Z, Evans A. Structural insights into aberrant topological patterns of large-scale cortical networks in Alzheimer's disease. J Neurosci. 2008;28(18):4756–66.

Hellwig B. A quantitative analysis of the local connectivity between pyramidal neurons in layers 2/3 of the rat visual cortex. Biol Cybern. 2000;82(2):111–21.

Hofbauer RK, Rainville P, Duncan GH, et al. Cortical representation of the sensory dimension of pain. J Neurophysiol. 2001;86:402–11.

Hoffman GA, Harrington A, Fields HL. Pain and the placebo: what we have learned. Perspect Biol Med. 2005;48:248–65.

Hsu CC, Weng CS, Sun MF, et al. Evaluation of scalp and auricular acupuncture on EEG, HRV, and PRV. Am J Chin Med. 2007;35:219–30.

Hui KK, Liu J, Makris N. Acupuncture modulates the limbic system and subcortical gray structures of the human brain: evidence from fMRI studies in normal subjects. Hum Brain Mapp. 2000;9:13–25.

Hui KK, Liu J, Marina O, et al. The integrated response of the human cerebro-cerebellar and limbic systems to acupuncture stimulation at ST 36 as evidenced by fMRI. NeuroImage. 2005;27:479–96.
Jeanette E, Brian B, Victoria AH, et al. Is acupuncture effective for the treatment of chronic pain? A systematic review. Pain. 2000;86:217–25.
Kamitani Y, Tong F. Decoding the visual and subjective contents of the human brain. Nat Neurosci. 2005;8(5):679–85.
Kaptchuk TJ. Acupuncture: theory, efficacy, and practice. Ann Intern Med. 2002;136:374–83.
Kong J, Ma L, Gollub RL, et al. A pilot study of functional magnetic resonance imaging of the brain during manual and electroacupuncture stimulation of acupuncture point (li-4 hegu) in normal subjects reveals differential brain activation between methods. J Altern Complement Med. 2002;8(7412):522–6.
Kong J, Randy LG, Webb JM, et al. Test-retest study of fMRI signal change evoked by electroacupuncture stimulation. NeuroImage. 2007;34:1171–81.
Kong J, Kaptchuk TJ, Webb JM, et al. Functional neuroanatomical investigation of vision-related acupuncture point specificity-a multisession fMRI study. Hum Brain Mapp. 2009;30(1):38–46.
Korte C, Milgram S. Acquaintance networks between racial groups: application of small-world method. J Pers Soc Psychol. 1970;15(2):101–8.
Kotter R. Neuroscience databases: tools for exploring brain structure-function relationships. Philos Trans R Soc Lond Ser B Biol Sci. 2001;356(1412):1111–20.
Latora V, Marchiori M. Efficient behavior of small-world networks. Phys Rev Lett. 2001;87(19):198701.
Latora V, Marchiori M. Economic small-world behavior in weighted networks. Eur Phys J B. 2003;32(2):249 63.
Le BD, Villanueva L, Willer J. Diffuse noxious inhibitory controls (DNIC) in animals and man. Acupunct Med. 1991;9:47–56.
Lindquist MA, Waugh C, Wager TD. Modeling state-related fMRI activity using change point theory. NeuroImage. 2007;35(3):1125–41.
Liu WC, Feldman SC, Cook DB, et al. fMRI study of acupuncture-induced periaqueductal gray activity in humans. Neuroreport. 2004;15:1937–40.
Liu Y, Liang M, Zhou Y, et al. Disrupted small-world networks in schizophrenia. Brain. 2008;131(4):945–61.
Liu JX, Liang JM, Qin W, et al. Dysfunctional connectivity patterns in chronic heroin users: an fMRI study. Neurosci Lett. 2009;460(1):72–7.
Liu J, Qin W, Guo Q. Distinct brain networks for time-varied characteristics of acupuncture. Neurosci Lett. 2010;468(3):353–8.
Lowe MJ, Mock BJ, Sorenson JA. Functional connectivity in single and multislice echo-planar imaging using resting-state fluctuations. NeuroImage. 1998;7(2):119–32.
MacPherson H, White A, Cummings M, et al. Standards for reporting interventions in controlled trials of acupuncture: the STRICTA recommendations. J Altern Complement Med. 2002;8(1):85–9.
Mann F. Reinventing acupuncture: a new concept of ancient medicine. Great Britain: Biddles Ltd.; 1992.
McKeown MJ, Makeig S, Brown GG, et al. Analysis of fMRI data by blind separation into independent spatial components. Hum Brain Mapp. 1998;6(3):160–88.
McIntosh AR, Gonzalez-Lima F. Structural equation modeling and its application to network analysis in functional brain imaging. Hum Brain Mapp. 1994;2(1–2):2–22.
Mechelli A, Price CJ, Noppeney U, et al. A dynamic causal modeling study on category effects: bottom-up or top-down mediation? J Cogn Neurosci. 2003;15(7):925–34.
Milgram S. Small-world problem. Psychol Today. 1967;1(1):61–7.
Millan MJ. Descending control of pain. Prog Neurobiol. 2002;66:355–474.
Mitchell TM, Hutchinson R, Niculescu RS, et al. Learning to decode cognitive states from brain images. Mach Learn. 2004;57(1–2):145–75.
Napadow V, Makris N, Liu J, et al. Effects of electroacupuncture versus manual acupuncture on the human brain as measured by fMRI. Hum Brain Mapp. 2005;24(3):193–205.

Napadow V, Liu J, Li M, et al. Somatosensory cortical plasticity in carpal tunnel syndrome treated by acupuncture. Hum Brain Mapp. 2007;30:38–46.

Napadow V, Dhond RP, Kim J, et al. Brain encoding of acupuncture sensation-coupling on-line rating with fMRI. NeuroImage. 2009a;47(3):1055–65.

Napadow V, Dhond R, Park K, et al. Time-variant fMRI activity in the brainstem and higher structures in response to acupuncture. NeuroImage. 2009b;47(1):289–301.

Newman ME. The structure and function of complex networks. SIAM Rev. 2003;45:167–256.

Norman KA, Polyn SM, Detre GJ, et al. Beyond mind-reading: multi-voxel pattern analysis of functional magnetic resonance imaging data. Trends Cogn Sci. 2006;10(9):424–30.

Oosterhof NN, Wiestler T, Downing PE, et al. A comparison of volume-based and surface-based multi-voxel pattern analysis. Neuroimage. 2011;56(2):593–600.

Pariente J, White P, Frackowiak RS, et al. Expectancy and belief modulate the neuronal substrates of pain treated by acupuncture. NeuroImage. 2005;25(4):1161–7.

Pastor-Satorras R, Vespignani A. Evolution and structure of the internet: a statistical physics approach. Cambridge: Cambridge University Press; 2004.

Peets JM, Pomeranz B. CXBK mice deficient in opiate receptors show poor electroacupuncture analgesia. Nature. 1978;273:675–6.

Pomeranz B. Acupuncture analgesia: basic research. In: Stux G, Hammerschlag R, editors. Clinical acupuncture: scientific basis. Berlin: Springer; 2001. p. 1–28.

Porreca F, Ossipov MH, Gebhart GF. Chronic pain and medullary descending facilitation. Trends Neurosci. 2002;25:319–25.

Price DD, Rafii A, Watkins LR. A psychophysical analysis of acupuncture analgesia. Pain. 1984;19:27–42.

Qin W, Tian J, Bai L. fMRI connectivity analysis of acupuncture effects on an amygdala associated brain network. Mol Pain. 2008;4:55.

Qin W, Bai L, Dai J. The temporal-spatial encoding of acupuncture effects in the brain. Mol Pain. 2011;7:19.

Rainville P, Duncan GH, Price DD, et al. Pain affect encoded in human anterior cingulate but not somatosensory cortex. Science. 1997;277:968–71.

Rainville P, Hofbauer RK, Paus T, et al. Cerebral mechanisms of hypnotic induction and suggestion. J Cogn Neurosci. 1999;11:110–25.

Reijneveld JC, Ponten SC, Berendse HW, et al. The application of graph theoretical analysis to complex networks in the brain. Clin Neurophysiol. 2007;118(11):2317–31.

Sakai S, Hori E, Umeno K, et al. Specific acupuncture sensation correlates with EEGs and autonomic changes in human subjects. Auton Neurosci. 2007;133:158–69.

Salvador R, Suckling J, Coleman MR, et al. Neurophysiological architecture of functional magnetic resonance images of human brain. Cereb Cortex. 2005;15(9):1332–42.

Siedentopf CM, Golaszewski SM, Mottaghy FM, et al. Functional magnetic resonance imaging detects activation of the visual association cortex during laser acupuncture of the foot in humans. Neurosci Lett. 2002;327(1):53–6.

Smith SM, Beckmann CF, Ramnani N, et al. Variability in fMRI: a re-examination of inter-session differences. Hum Brain Mapp. 2005;24:248–57.

Sporns O, Tononi G, Edelman GM. Theoretical neuroanatomy: relating anatomical and functional connectivity in graphs and cortical connection matrices. Cereb Cortex. 2000;10(2):127–41.

Stanley HE. Introduction to phase transitions and critical phenomena. New York: Oxford University Press; 1971.

Streitberger K, Kleinhenz J. Introducing a placebo needle into acupuncture research. Lancet. 1998;352:364–5.

Supekar K, Menon V, Rubin D, et al. Network analysis of intrinsic functional brain connectivity in Alzheimer's disease. PLoS Comput Biol. 2008;4(6):e1000100.

Takeda W, Wessel J. Acupuncture for the treatment of pain of osteoarthritic knees. Arthritis Care Res. 1994;7(3):118–22.

Tortorici V, Vanegas H. Putative role of medullary off- and on-cells in the antinociception produced by dipyrone (metamizol) administered systemically or microinjected into PAG. Pain. 1994;57:197–205.

Travers J, Milgram S. Experimental study of small-world problem. Sociometry. 1969;32(4):425–43.

Urban MO, Gebhart GF. Supraspinal contributions to hyperalgesia. Proc Nat Acad Sci U S A. 1999;96:7687–92.

van den Heuvel MP, Stam CJ, Boersma M, et al. Small-world and scale-free organization of voxel-based resting-state functional connectivity in the human brain. NeuroImage. 2008;43(3):528–39.

Wager TD, Vazquez A, Hernandez L. Accounting for nonlinear BOLD effects in fMRI: parameter estimates and a model for prediction in rapid event-related studies. NeuroImage. 2005;25(1):206–18.

Wang L, Zhu CZ, He Y, et al. Altered small-world brain functional networks in children with attention-deficit/hyperactivity disorder. Hum Brain Mapp. 2009;30(2):638–49.

Wang L, Li Y, Metzak P, et al. Age-related changes in topological patterns of large-scale brain functional networks during memory encoding and recognition. NeuroImage. 2010;50(3):862–72.

Watts DJ. Small worlds: the dynamics of networks between order and randomness. Princeton: Princeton University Press; 1999.

Watts DJ, Strogatz SH. Collective dynamics of 'small-world' networks. Nature. 1998;393(6684):440–2.

White A, Foster NE, Cummings M, et al. Acupuncture treatment for chronic knee pain: a systematic review. Rheumatology. 2007;46:384–90.

Witt C, Brinkhaus B, Jena S, et al. Acupuncture in patients with osteoarthritis of the knee: a randomised trial. Lancet. 2005;366:136–43.

Worsley KJ, Friston KJ. Analysis of fMRI time-series revisited again. NeuroImage. 1995;2(3):173–81.

Wu MT, Hsieh JC, Xiong J, et al. Central nervous pathway for acupuncture stimulation: localization of processing with functional MR imaging of the brain—preliminary experience. Radiology. 1999;212:133–41.

Wu MT, Sheen JM, Chuang KH, et al. Neuronal specificity of acupuncture response: a fMRI study with electroacupuncture. NeuroImage. 2002;16:1028–37.

Xing GG, Liu FY, XX Q, et al. Long-term synaptic plasticity in the spinal dorsal horn and its modulation by electroacupuncture in rats with neuropathic pain. J Pharmacol Exp Ther. 2007;321:1046–53.

Yan B, Li K, Xu J, et al. Acupoint-specific fMRI patterns in human brain. Neurosci Lett. 2005;383(3):236–40.

Yoo SS, Teh EK, Blinder RA, et al. Modulation of cerebellar activities by acupuncture stimulation: evidence from fMRI study. NeuroImage. 2004;22:932–40.

Zhang WT, Jin Z, Cui GH, et al. Relations between brain network activation and analgesic effect induced by low vs. high frequency electrical acupoint stimulation in different subjects: a functional magnetic resonance imaging study. Brain Res. 2003;982:168–78.

Zhang Y, Qin W, Liu P, et al. An fMRI study of acupuncture using independent component analysis. Neurosci Lett. 2009;449(1):6–9.

Targeting Mechanisms of Typical Indications of Acupuncture

3

Zhenyu Liu, Zhenchao Tang, and Jie Tian

3.1 Introduction

As described in the 2011 White Paper of Society of Acupuncture Research, "one of the bottlenecks in current studies on the acupuncture mechanism is the gap between basic research and clinical research." This gap is particularly obvious in neuroimaging studies of the central mechanism of acupuncture. Between 1998 and 2011, only nine studies were published that focused on mechanisms of disease with respect to acupuncture, which is less than 10% of the number of studies conducted using healthy subjects. In addition, controversial or contradictory findings are often reported in studies that use different models of diseases. Given the utility of disease biomarkers in the brain in previous studies, and that acupuncture is known to have regulatory effects on the brain for the treatment of some diseases, it can be proposed that the target of acupuncture and central biomarkers of diseases may converge in the same spatial location.

In this chapter, we explore the researches focusing on central biomarkers of disease as a priori information to explore the central mechanisms of acupuncture. These studies focus on the pathologies of heroin addiction, Internet addiction, and migraine and utilized multi-model data analysis methods, incorporating both spatial and temporal brain activity information. The findings showed alterations in the resting-state brain network and brain structure (in gray and white matter) in models of addiction, migraine, and functional dyspepsia and ultimately informed the utility and mechanisms of acupuncture treatment.

Z. Liu • Z. Tang • J. Tian (✉)
CAS Key Laboratory of Molecular Imaging, Institute of Automation, Beijing, China
e-mail: jie.tian@ia.ac.cn

© Springer Nature Singapore Pte Ltd. 2018

J. Tian (ed.), *Multi-Modality Neuroimaging Study on Neurobiological Mechanisms of Acupuncture*, DOI 10.1007/978-981-10-4914-9_3

3.2 Mechanisms of Addiction

Drug addiction is defined as compulsively taking drugs and leading to complex interactions between biological and environmental variables (Goldstein and Volkow 2002). With the advancement of medical advancement, there have been many scientific breakthroughs on the mechanisms of drug addiction. Heroin addiction is a complex disease of affective and cognitive processes in the brain (Buttner et al. 2000; Goldstein and Volkow 2002). There have been numerous previous imaging studies revealing that drug addiction would bring about neurochemical and functional changes in the brains. These studies have provided understanding of the underlying mechanisms of disease (Shalev et al. 2002; Li and Sinha 2008). In previous studies, increased white matter intensity in the frontal area and decreased gray matter density in the bilateral prefrontal cortices and temporal regions were observed among heroin-dependent individuals (Lyoo et al. 2004, 2006; Yuan et al. 2009). Accordingly, functional impairments have been identified in individuals with heroin addiction in a variety of tasks, such as response inhibition and decision-making (Lee et al. 2005; Xiao et al. 2006; Fu et al. 2008).

3.2.1 Alterations in Resting-State Functional Connectivity in Heroin Addiction

Heroin addiction demonstrated cue reactivity, which caused significant psychophysiological reactions. Previous studies of cue reactivity found that addicts have significant cue-specific reactions to drug-related stimuli. Previous studies found that the drug-related cue activation was related to brain circuits and had an effect on the decision-making, inhibitory control, stress regulation, and emotional valence assignment (Sinha 2001; Lee and Pau 2002; Lee et al. 2005). However, the exact mechanisms underlying these alterations in heroin addiction are not fully understood. In a cue-related previous study, Liu et al. explored the regional brain activity in chronic heroin users and found dysfunctional connectivity in memory, inhibition, and motivation-related dysfunctions during a resting state free of cues (Liu et al. 2009). In this study, the brain regional interactions of 12 chronic heroin users and 12 control subjects were compared with a novel graph theory analysis (GTA) method. First, fMRI data divided into 90 regions of interest (ROIs) was registered to an anatomically labeled template image used previously by Tzourio-Mazoyer and colleagues (2002). By averaging the fMRI time series of all voxels in each ROI over the entire brain, regional mean time series were extracted. Partial correlations were used to construct undirected graphs, and the edges between regional nodes represented the whole-brain functional network. A graph was defined as having 90 nodes (in this study, ROIs) and edges (functional connections). Liu et al. obtained topological maps for brain functional networks during the resting state from non-drug users and chronic heroin users (Fig. 3.1). In comparison with non-drug users, chronic heroin users had significantly higher connectivity strength in the anterior cingulate cortex (ACC), supramarginal motor area, hippocampus, amygdala, insula, putamen, pallidum, caudate, dorsolateral superior frontal gyrus, and orbital inferior frontal gyrus.

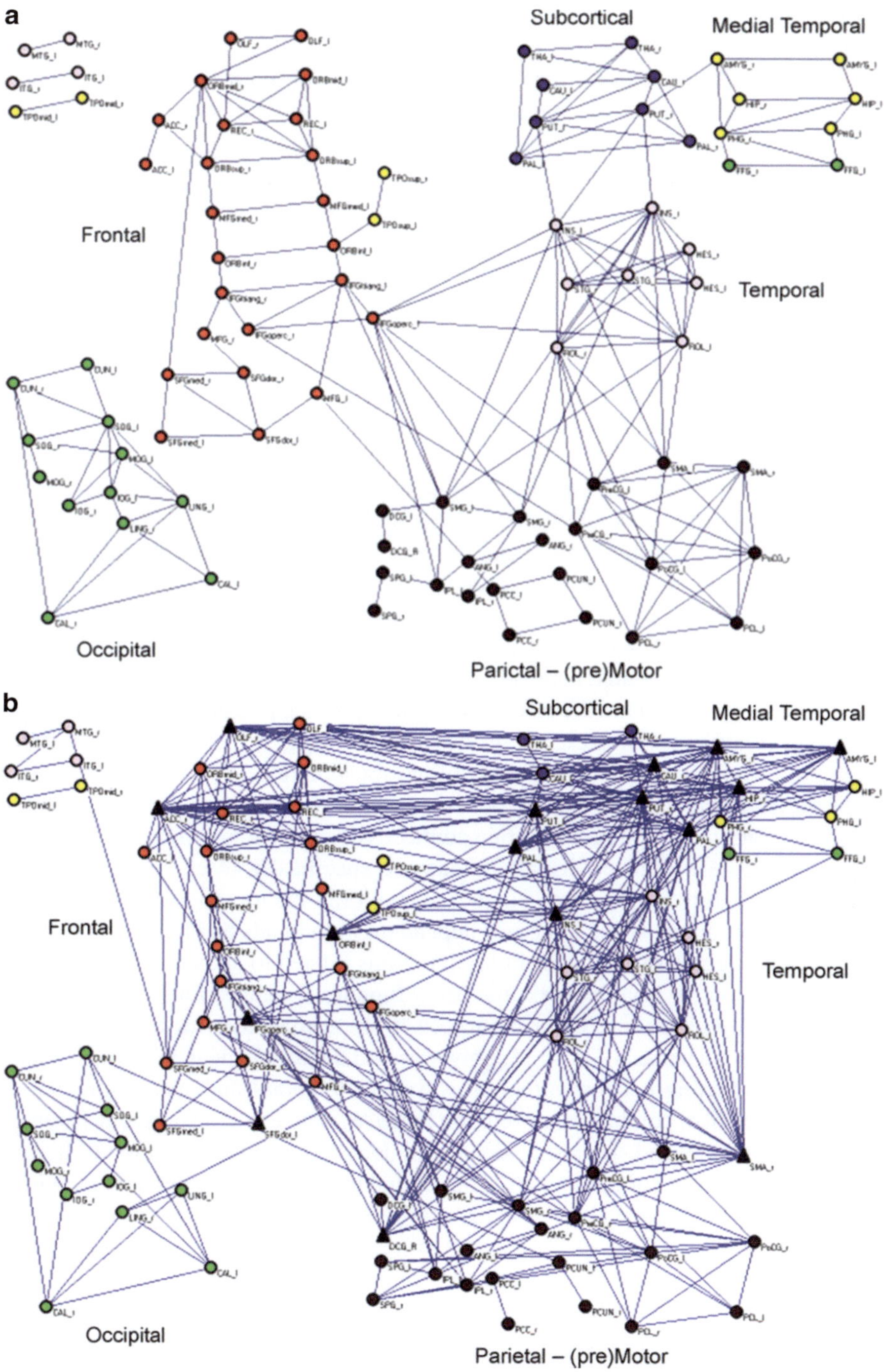

Fig. 3.1 The topological map of non-drug users (**a**) and chronic heroin users (**b**) (Reprint with permission from Liu et al. 2009). The colors represented medial temporal (*yellow*), subcortical (*purple*), temporal (*pink*), parietal-(pre)motor (*brown*), frontal (*red*), and occipital (*green*). *Black triangles* represent the most remarkable increases in connectivity strength in chronic heroin users versus non-drug users ($P < 0.05$, two-sample t-test) (Liu et al. 2009)

As shown in Fig. 3.1, dysfunctional integrations were detected among the heroin-addicted individuals during the resting state. Repeated drug administration might lead to significant alterations in dendritic branching and spine density resultant and pathway irregularities in chronic heroin user, which subsequently led to irregular brain network connectivity and the abovementioned cognitive impairments.

3.2.1.1 Alterations in Functional Network Characteristics According to Duration of Heroin Use

Several recent studies investigated the human brain's resting-state networks (Greicius et al. 2003; Fox and Raichle 2007; Buckner et al. 2008) and found that the correlated spontaneous activity occured during task-free conditions (Greicius et al. 2003; Ma et al. 2010). It was also found that the BOLD (Blood Oxygenation Level Dependent) signal fluctuations occur at low frequencies (0.01–0.08 Hz) (Fox and Raichle 2007). In addition, the resting-state networks in brain disorders were assessed at the level of systems integration during task-free conditions (Wang et al. 2006; Garrity et al. 2007). Further, resting-state fMRI is a validated approach for the study of disease. In previous studies, it was found that the decreased connectivity between the hippocampus and visual cortices has been observed in Alzheimer's disease (AD) and abnormal resting-state bilateral frontoparietal, fronto-cingulate, and fronto-thalamic connectivity was observed in schizophrenia patients. The findings in previous studies revealed the pathological alterations in the integrity and efficiency of disease-related networks (Wang et al. 2006; Garrity et al. 2007). These findings help to understand the disease states and provide potential diagnostic information or treatment strategies. All of these studies suggest that resting-state fMRI might be a useful approach to the study of heroin addiction.

In previous studies, Liu et al. (2009) and Ma et al. (2010) observed addiction-related alterations in resting-state brain connectivity, while it is still unclear whether these resting-state connectivity alterations are specifically to chronic heroin use (Yuan et al. 2010a). In contrast, Yuan et al. explored the topological properties of resting-state brain networks in heroin-dependent individuals and hypothesized that network disruptions would occur in brain regions related to addictive behavior and stress regulation. In Yuan's work, the brain functional connections of the heroin-dependent individuals and control subjects were compared with a graph theory analysis (GTA). This analysis thoroughly assessed the topological properties of networks by evaluating network strength as well as temporal and spatial interaction patterns. They also conducted correlation analyses between the statistical parameters (the degree, D, and shortest absolute path length, L) and the duration of heroin use in heroin-dependent individuals. They found that in heroin-dependent individuals, D values were higher in the bilateral orbitofrontal cortex (OFC), dorsolateral prefrontal cortex (PFC), rostral ACC (rACC), precuneus, parahippocampal gyrus, putamen, and cerebellum; the left inferior frontal cortex, medial PFC, caudate, thalamus, and posterior cingulate cortex (PCC); and finally, the right middle temporal gyrus relative to control subjects (Fig. 3.2). Moreover, they observed positive correlation between the duration of heroin and the D value in the right parahippocampal gyrus, left putamen, and bilateral cerebellum. It was also observed that the

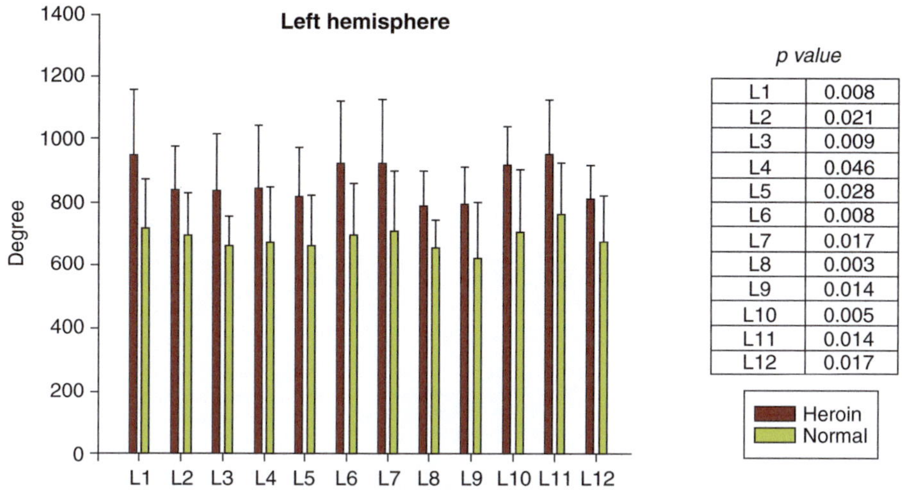

L1	0.008
L2	0.021
L3	0.009
L4	0.046
L5	0.028
L6	0.008
L7	0.017
L8	0.003
L9	0.014
L10	0.005
L11	0.014
L12	0.017

L1. Cerebellum L2. Inferior Frontal Gyrus L3. Medial Prefrontal Cortex L4. Orbitofrontal Cortex L5. Dorsolateral Prefrontal Cortex L6. Anterior Cingulate Cortex L7. Parahippocam Gyrus L8. Posterior Cingulate Cortex L9. Precuneus L10. Caudate L11. Putamen L12. Thalamus

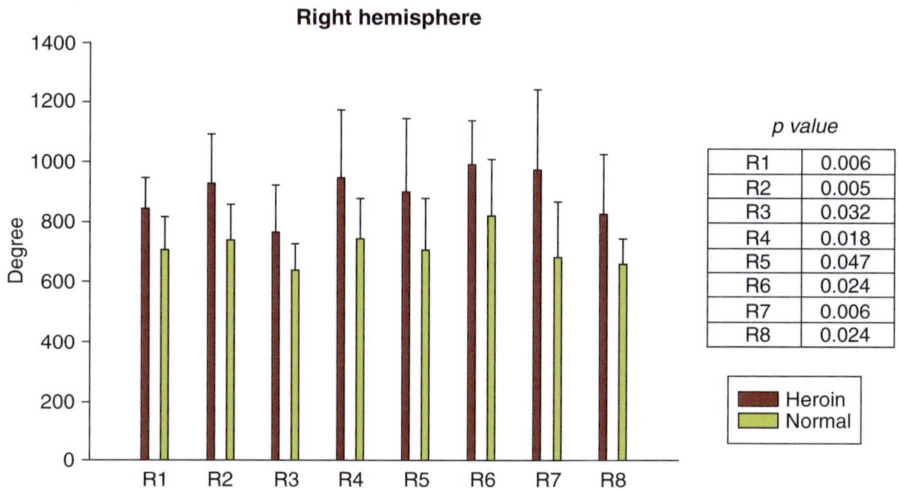

R1	0.006
R2	0.005
R3	0.032
R4	0.018
R5	0.047
R6	0.024
R7	0.006
R8	0.024

R1. Cerebellum R2. Dorsolateral Prefrontal Cortex R3. Orbitofrontal Cortex R4. Anterior Cingulate Cortex R5. Parahippocampal Gyrus R6. Putamen R7. Middle temporal gyrus R8. Precuneus

Fig. 3.2 The degrees of chronic heroin users were different from the control subjects (Reprint with permission from Yuan et al. 2010a)

duration of heroin use was negatively correlated with the L parameter in the same regions ($P < 0.05$) (Fig. 3.3).

The areas of elevated D values in heroin-dependent patients were distributed in addiction-related circuits: the caudate and putamen of the reward circuit; the OFC

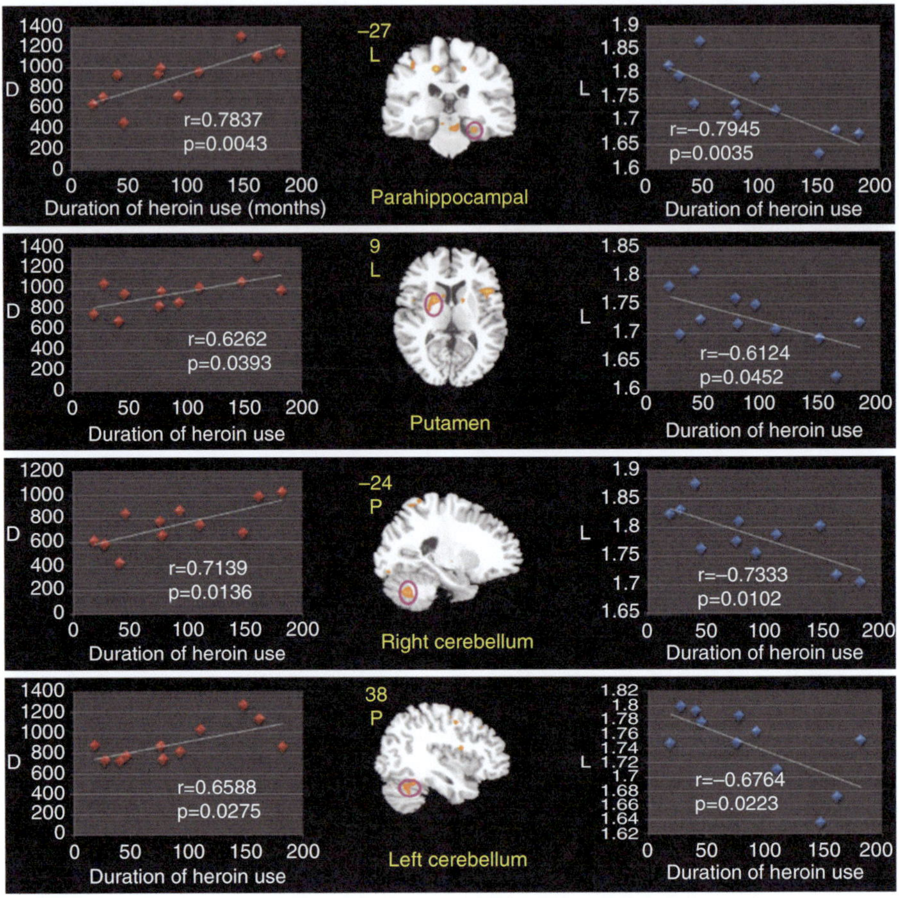

Fig. 3.3 The duration of heroin use was correlated with the regional topological properties (D value and L parameter) (Reprint with permission from Yuan et al. 2010a)

and dorsolateral PFC of motivation/drive circuitry; the parahippocampal gyrus involved in memory; the rACC of the control circuit, consistent with a previous study (Fu et al. 2008); and the medial PFC representing stress regulation and emotional modulation. The findings of the abnormal topological properties might help to understand the underlying mechanism of heroin addiction.

The dorsolateral PFC integrates cognitive and motivational information from the OFC and contributes to regulatory processing (Groenewegen and Uylings 2000). In addition, there are studies which found that the OFC and dorsolateral PFC were important in the motivation-relevant processes of drug addiction (Goldstein and Volkow 2002; Goldstein et al. 2007). The parahippocampal gyrus is very important for memory encoding and retrieval. Memory is likely to influence the effects of drug use during intoxication (Shalev et al. 2002; Volkow et al. 2003). In addition, this area may be related to cue reactivity as mentioned earlier, where places, people, or other cues trigger an intense desire for drug use (Shalev et al. 2002). In previous heroin studies, hypoactivation of the rACC has been reported (control circuit) in heroin users (Fu et al. 2008) and cocaine users (Kaufman et al. 2003) during a GO/NOGO task, which indicated a role for the rACC in inhibitory control. Accordingly, the alterations observed in the work of Yuan et al. are consistent with what is known regarding the neurobiological basis of addiction and further inform the interconnectivity of relevant regions.

Yuan also found that the duration of heroin use is related to the topological properties (D and L) of several brain regions, including the bilateral cerebellum, right parahippocampal gyrus, and left putamen. The results suggest that heroin use has a cumulative effect on brain topology. An interesting interpretation of this result is that the information transfer of reward and memory becomes progressively more complicated with prolonged heroin use and probably leads to poor control and decision-making. These results agreed with a previous behavioral study which observed that the duration of heroin use was correlated to the performance in a stop-signal task (Monterosso et al. 2005). It can be concluded that the early intervention was crucial for the treatment of heroin addiction.

3.2.1.2 Spatial and Temporal Alterations in Resting-State Networks Related to Heroin Addiction

In Yuan's work, spatial and temporal information was combined to investigate the resting-state networks changes in heroin-dependent individuals (Yuan et al. 2010b). In their work, the relationship between resting-state functional connectivity changes and duration of heroin use was investigated with correlation analysis. Yuan et al. employed the discrete cosine transform (DCT) (Fransson 2005) to assess the spatial distribution of low-frequency BOLD oscillations during resting state between the heroin-dependent individuals and healthy subjects. In addition, the temporal characteristics of brain regions that exhibited similar spatial patterns in DCT analysis were also investigated between the heroin-dependent individuals and healthy subjects. It was assumed that the resting-state functional connectivity of heroin-dependent individuals was changed and was correlated with duration of heroin use.

In comparison with healthy subjects, widespread spontaneous fluctuations in the resting state were detected in heroin-dependent individuals. Spontaneous signal changes were mainly found in the regions including posterior cingulate cortex (PCC)/precuneus, ACC, inferior parietal lobe, supplementary motor area (SMA), middle temporal lobe, and occipital lobe in heroin-dependent individuals and healthy subjects (Fig. 3.4).

In a later study, Fransson and Marrelec applied a partial correlation analysis and found that out of all the regions in the default mode network (DMN), the PCC/precuneus was the only region connected with all other regions (Fransson and Marrelec 2008). The findings of Fransson and Marrelec might suggest that the PCC/precuneus played an important role in the DMN. Accordingly, in the work of Yuan, the PCC/precuneus was selected as the ROI to detect alterations in the PCC/precuneus network among the heroin-dependent individuals. In comparison, significantly reduced functional connectivity between the PCC/precuneus and right cerebellum

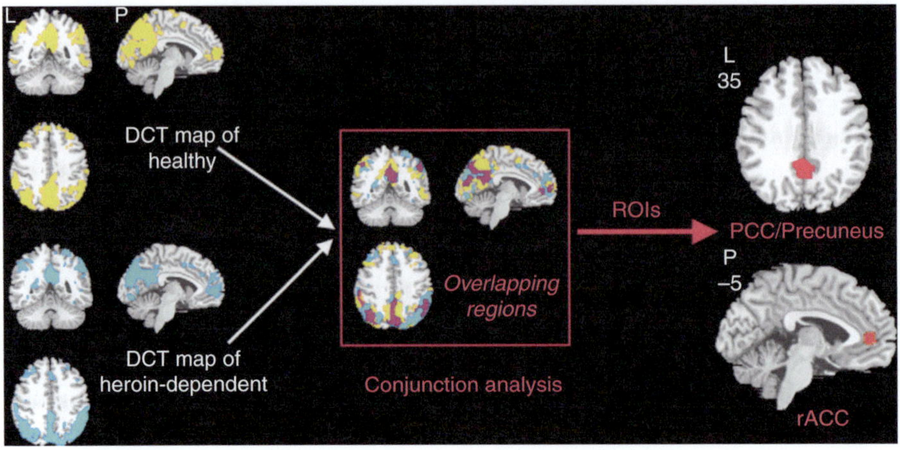

Fig. 3.4 Discrete cosine transform analysis result (Reprint with permission from Yuan et al. 2010b). The regions of interest for the functional connectivity analysis (PCC/precuneus and rACC) were chosen from overlapping regions between heroin-dependent individuals and healthy subjects

($P < 0.05$, corrected) was found among the heroin-dependent individuals. They also found that the resting-state functional connectivity between the PCC/precuneus and right cerebellum was negatively correlated with duration of heroin use in heroin-dependent individuals (Fig. 3.4). In conclusion, the DMN was thought to facilitate the retrieval and manipulation of past events for decision-making (Greicius et al. 2003), and it might be inferred that the decreased functional connectivity between the PCC/precuneus and right cerebellum in the DMN may have an effect on the decision-making in heroin-dependent patients.

3.2.1.3 Gray Matter Loss and Resting-State Abnormalities in Abstinent Heroin-Dependent Individuals

There have been only few studies investigating the gray matter density and the resting-state functional connectivity changes of heroin-dependent individuals. In the previous study, Yuan employed the voxel-based morphometry (VBM) to identify the decreased gray matter density in heroin-dependent individuals (Yuan et al. 2010c). In addition, Yuan also investigated the altered functional connectivity on resting-state fMRI among the heroin-dependent individuals (Yuan et al. 2010c). In comparison with the healthy control, significant reductions in gray matter density in the right dorsolateral PFC, left IPL, right fusiform gyrus, and left middle cingulate cortex (MCC) were observed among the heroin-dependent individuals (Fig. 3.5a). No significant increases in gray matter density were found. Moreover, it was found that the gray matter density of the right dorsolateral PFC was negatively correlated ($r = -0.8359$, $P = 0.0013$) with the duration of heroin use in heroin-dependent individuals (Fig. 3.5b).

In healthy subjects, activity in several brain regions was positively correlated with that in the right dorsolateral PFC, including the bilateral insula, putamen,

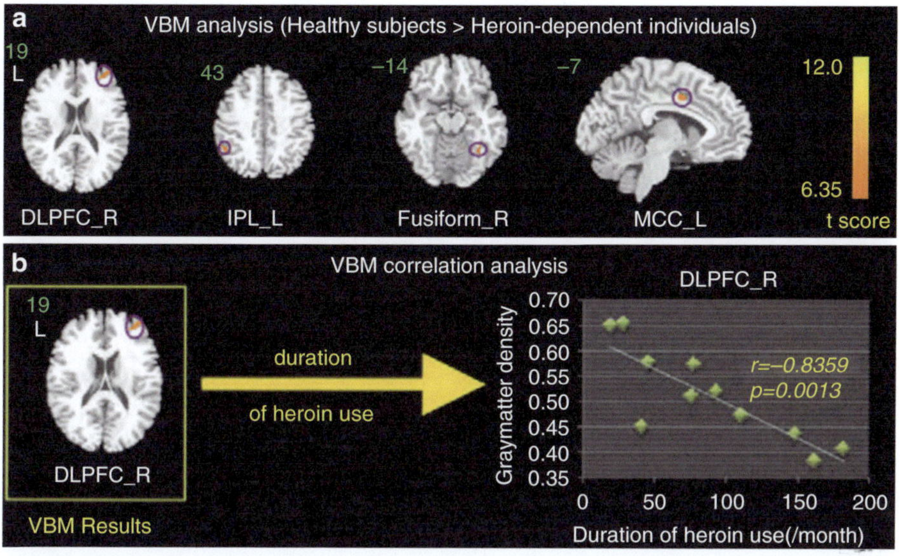

Fig. 3.5 Voxel-based morphometry (VBM) analysis results (Reprint with permission from Yuan et al. 2010c). (**a**) The VBM analysis (**b**) correlation analysis results (*r*, correlation coefficient; *p*, *P*-value). *DLPFC* dorsolateral prefrontal cortex, *IPL* inferior parietal lobe, *L* left, *MCC* middle cingulate cortex, *R* right

caudate, MCC, IPL, ACC, and OFC, and the right thalamus and fusiform gyrus ($P < 0.05$, family-wise error rate [FWER] corrected). However, in heroin-dependent individuals, activity in the right insula, MCC, fusiform gyrus, and IPL was positively correlated with that in the right dorsolateral PFC ($P < 0.05$, FWER corrected). In comparison with the healthy subjects, significantly reduced functional connectivity between the right dorsolateral PFC and bilateral IPL ($P < 0.05$, corrected) was observed among the heroin-dependent individuals ($P < 0.05$, corrected) (Fig. 3.6a). It was also found that the functional connectivity between the right dorsolateral PFC and left IPL was significantly negatively correlated with the duration of heroin use ($r = -0.7676$, $P = 0.0058$) (Fig. 3.6b).

The findings in the abovementioned study were consistent with previous studies (Lyoo et al. 2006; Yuan et al. 2009). Furthermore, a negative relationship between the gray matter density of the right dorsolateral PFC and the duration of heroin use further confirmed a cumulative effect of heroin use on the brain in an addiction-related region. Numerous studies have indicated that drug-related cues elicit significant activation of the dorsolateral PFC in users (Garavan et al. 2000; Bonson et al. 2002; Due et al. 2002). As indicated in previous study, the neurons in the dorsolateral PFC encoded reward expectancy during a delay, which was very important for the subsequent behavioral responses in rewarded tasks (Wallis and Miller 2003). It was also found that the impairments of the rat prelimbic cortex would hamper the acquisition and modification of contingency-guided behavior, indicating that this region is crucial for the cognitive control of goal-directed behavior (Balleine and

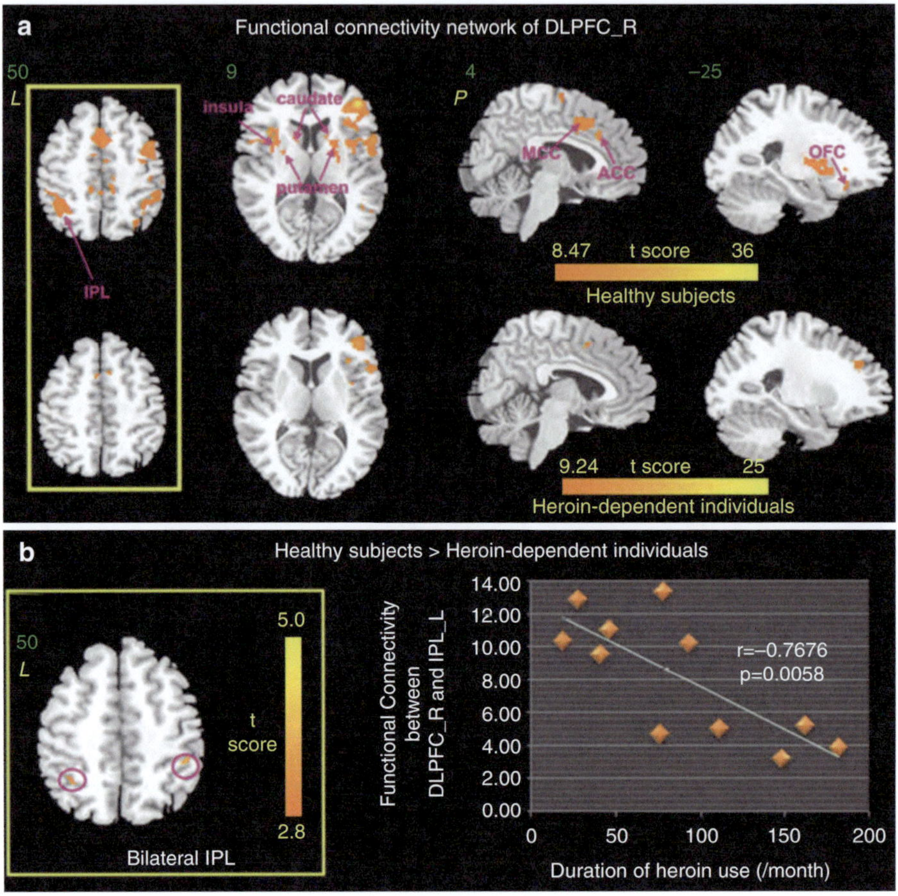

Fig. 3.6 Functional connectivity network results (Reprint with permission from Yuan et al. 2010c). (**a**) The connectivities of right dorsolateral prefrontal cortex and (**b**) the connectivities of heroin-dependent individuals were different from healthy subjects ($P < 0.05$, corrected). The correlation analysis was shown in the lower panel (r, correlation coefficient; p, P-value). *ACC* anterior cingulate cortex, *DLPFC* dorsolateral prefrontal cortex, *IPL* inferior parietal lobe, *L* left, *MCC* middle cingulate cortex, *OFC* orbital frontal cortex, *P* posterior, *R* right

Dickinson 1998). In the previous study, the dorsolateral PFC was found crucial for the decision-making tasks requiring the integration of cognitive and motivationally relevant information (Wilson et al. 2004). Thus, reduced gray matter intensity in the dorsolateral PFC was likely in part associated with impaired decision-making and goal-directed behavior dysfunction in heroin dependence (Lyoo et al. 2006; Xiao et al. 2006; Ma et al. 2010).

Several studies have reported that the IPL also integrated information from different sensory modalities to participate in higher cognitive functions (Caspers et al. 2006). For both humans and animals, the bilateral IPL is activated during working memory paradigms (Greicius et al. 2003). In addition, Park et al. reported significant activation in the bilateral IPL and right fusiform gyrus in response to alcohol-related cues among subjects with alcohol use disorders (Park et al. 2007). In the work by Yuan, the functional connectivity between the right dorsolateral PFC and bilateral IPL was found significantly decreased when compared with healthy control. In addition, the functional connectivity between the right dorsolateral PFC and left IPL was significantly negatively correlated with the duration of heroin use. These results suggested that persistent heroin use progressively degrades communication between the right dorsolateral PFC and left IPL in a manner possibly related to reported functional impairments in decision-making and cognitive control in these individuals (Xiao et al. 2006; Fu et al. 2008). It was also observed that the gray matter changes in the right dorsolateral PFC agreed with the resting-state functional connectivity alterations among the abstinent heroin-dependent individuals, which might indicate that the alteration in functional connectivity was of systems level (Xiao et al. 2006; Fu et al. 2008). While, it was noteworthy that the relationship of gray matter density changes to functional connectivity was still unclear. In the future, more work is needed to explore this issue.

3.2.2 Microstructural Abnormalities in Adolescents with Internet Addiction Disorder (IAD)

Worldwide use of the Internet has expanded incredibly in the last decade. The Internet provides remote access to other individuals and abundant information in all areas of interest. The IAD has been more and more prevalent and becomes serious society problem, which has attracted the attention of psychiatrists, educators, and the public. Due to the reason that the cognitive control and the impulse control of adolescents are relatively immature, they are at a high risk for addiction problems such as IAD. Though there have been studies suggesting that the IAD was related to gray matter changes, there have been few studies investigating the microstructural integrity of major neuronal fiber pathways in IAD, and almost no studies to date have assessed the temporal course of these changes.

In a more recent study, Yuan and colleagues used an optimized VBM method to investigate brain morphology in adolescents with IAD according to disease duration (Yuan et al. 2011). From previous studies, it was known that IAD subjects showed impaired cognitive control, and accordingly the authors hypothesized that long-term IAD would result in structural alterations in the brain associated with cognitive functional impairment. Assessing regional gray matter volume changes nonparametrically with an optimized VBM method and correcting for multiple comparisons using a cluster-based thresholding method, it was determined that IAD subjects had decreased gray matter volume in several clusters relative to matched control subjects; these regions were the bilateral dorsolateral PFC, SMA, OFC, cerebellum, and left rACC. Moreover, gray matter volumes of the right dorsolateral PFC, left rACC, and right SMA showed significant negative correlations with disease duration ($r_1 = 20.73$, $P_1 < 0.005$; $r_2 = 20.74$, $P_2 < 0.005$; $r_3 = 20.65$, $P_3 = 0.005$). No brain regions showed higher gray matter volumes with respect to matched control subjects (Fig. 3.7).

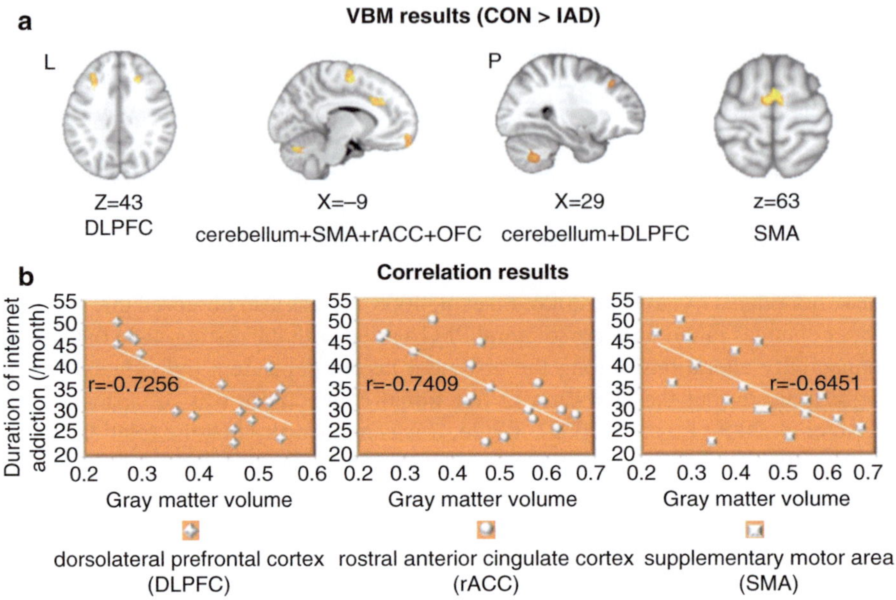

Fig. 3.7 Voxel-based morphometry results (Reprint from Yuan et al. 2011). (**a**) The gray matter volume of subjects with Internet addiction disorder (IAD) was reduced when compared to the control subjects. (**b**) Gray matter volumes of the dorsolateral prefrontal cortex (DLPFC), rostral anterior cingulate cortex (rACC), and supplementary motor area (SMA) were negatively correlated with duration of Internet addiction

As indicated in previous studies, long-term substance abuse (Kaufman et al. 2003; Li and Sinha 2008) and Internet addiction (Zhou et al. 2011) would bring about the cognitive control impairments. Numerous functional neuroimaging studies have revealed that the dorsolateral PFC and rACC were centrally involved in cognitive control as components of a specific cortico-subcortical circuit (MacDonald et al. 2000; Krawczyk 2002; Wilson et al. 2004). It was hypothesized that the occurrence of response conflict was signaled by the rACC, which would recruit the dorsolateral PFC for improved cognitive control. This important role of the dorsolateral PFC has been identified as an important top-down regulatory process (Vanderhasselt et al. 2009). In support of these hypotheses, recent neuroimaging studies have reported deactivation of the rACC in heroin and cocaine users during a GO/NOGO task (Fu et al. 2008; Vanderhasselt et al. 2009).

The OFC played an important role in the assessment of motivational significance for a given stimulus and the selection of behavior to obtain a desired outcome and contributes to the cognitive control of goal-directed behavior. For the reason that the OFC was extensively connected with the striatum and limbic regions (such as the amygdala), the OFC was suitable to integrate the activity of several limbic and subcortical areas associated with motivational behavior and reward processing (Groenewegen and Uylings 2000). As indicated in previous animal studies, the damage of OFC or the rat prelimbic would impair contingency-guided behavior, which might indicate that these regions are crucial for the cognitive control of goal-directed behavior. The SMA was critical for the selection of an appropriate behavior or inhibition of an inappropriate response. Indeed, the reported role of the SMA in both simple and complex GO/NOGO tasks suggested its importance in mediating cognitive control (Li et al. 2006; Li and Sinha 2008).

3.3 Mechanisms of Migraine

Migraine is an idiopathic headache disorder that is a significant source of individual and social burden and can lead to disability, losses of productivity, and a decreased overall quality of life (Terwindt et al. 2000; Li et al. 2006; Schwedt and Dodick 2009). Migraine attacks furthermore increase the risk of developing brain lesions in some regions (Tietjen 2004; Zaidat 2004). Recently, research interest has been directed toward the CNS damage and dysregulation associated with headaches and migraine. With the development of neuroimaging technology, the mechanism of migraine has transformed from a vascular disorder to a neurovascular disorder and, finally, to a central nervous system disorder (Schwedt and Dodick 2009). Accordingly, advanced neuroimaging approaches have been employed to investigate the structural and functional changes occurring in migraine patients (May 2009a; Schwedt and Dodick 2009).

3.3.1 Regional Homogeneity Abnormalities in Patients with Interictal Migraine

As indicated in previous studies, migraine without aura would lead to structural and task-related functional changes in the brains. While resting-state brain studies in particular have the utility to inform the pathophysiology of migraine, there have been only few studies focusing on the resting-state abnormalities in patients with migraine without aura. In the work of Yu, the local features of spontaneous brain activity in patients with migraine without aura were analyzed by the regional homogeneity (ReHo) method (Yu et al. 2012). Firstly, one-sample t-test was used to extract the ReHo results across all the subjects. Then, two-sample *t*-test was applied to compare ReHo between the patients with migraine without aura group and the healthy control group ($P < 0.05$, FWE corrected). Yu observed significantly decreased ReHo values in the right rACC, PFC, OFC, and SMA in the patients with migraine without aura when compared with ($P < 0.05$, FWE corrected). In the correlation analysis, the duration of migraine was found significantly negatively correlated with the average ReHo values in the right PFC ($r = -0.5032$, $P = 0.0088$) and rACC ($r = -0.4306$, $P = 0.0281$) (Fig. 3.8). However, no relationships were found between resting-state properties and the average pain intensity or attack frequency in migraine patients.

Both experimental and clinical studies have suggested that affective responses to pain such as unpleasantness and suffering were principally integrated in the rACC

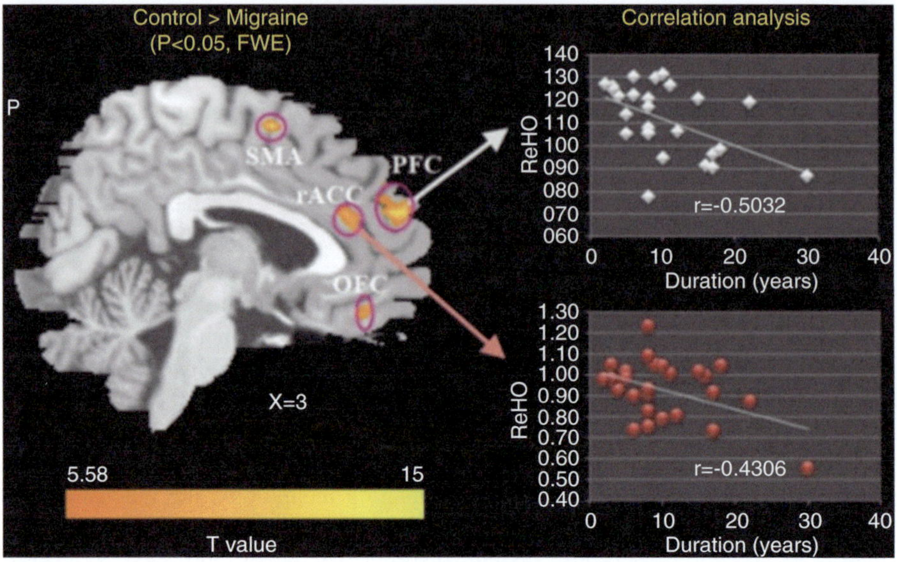

Fig. 3.8 Altered regional homogeneity in migraine (Reprint with permission from Yu et al. 2012). (*Left*) Migraine-related changes in regional homogeneity (ReHo) shown as a comparison of Kendall's coefficient of concordance (KCC) maps between patients with migraine without aura and control subjects ($P < 0.05$, corrected) during the resting state. (*Right*) The average ReHo values of the right prefrontal cortex (PFC) were significantly correlated to the disease duration

(Vogt 2005; Mechias et al. 2010; Shackman et al. 2011). In addition, the rACC was involved in pain control mediated by the endogenous opioid system (Petrovic et al. 2002; Wager et al. 2004). It might be inferred that the functional disruption in the rACC of patients with migraine without aura might be the underlying mechanism of the functional impairments in long-term pain affective responses and endogenous analgesia.

The PFC was another important region in opioid analgesia and other forms of pain modulation (Kupers et al. 2000; Petrovic et al. 2002). In particular, the PFC may play a role in suppressing pain perception via cognitive control mechanisms (Lieberman et al. 2004; Wiech et al. 2008). Aderjan et al. used fMRI to study the differences between the patients and healthy control subjects stimulated daily with trigeminal pain, 20 min per day for 8 consecutive days. The fMRI was obtained in day 1, day 8, and 3 months later. No difference on the behavioral pain ratings was observed between the two groups. While, they found opposing activity changes in several brain regions involved in endogenous pain control. The brain activity in PFC and rACC was found increased in healthy control subjects while decreased in the patients with migraine. The findings might indicate reduced efficiency in pain processing in patients with migraine without aura. In the correlation analysis, they also found that negative relationship between the ReHo values in the rACC and PFC and the duration of disease.

As indicated in previous studies, the OFC was involved in the behavior associated with sensitivity to reward and punishment, including sensory integration, decision-making, expectation, and planning (Bechara et al. 1994). Both positive (pleasure) and negative (pain) stimulation has been shown to elicit opioid release in the OFC (Phillips et al. 2003). Accordingly, all received sensations were likely to be modulated and assigned affective responses by the OFC (Vincent et al. 2003). In particular, the OFC seemed to be related to the responses based on the previous reward value need to be inhibited (Elliott et al. 2000). Similarly, the SMA seemed to be crucial for linking cognition to action (Picard and Strick 1996; Rushworth et al. 2004). The pre-SMA was involved in executive control (Curtis et al. 2005; Nachev et al. 2005; Aron and Poldrack 2006; Li et al. 2006), pain anticipation (Ploghaus et al. 1999; Wager et al. 2004; Roy et al. 2009), and the affective component of pain (Apkarian et al. 2005). The pre-SMA was also activated in the tasks requiring the inhibition of responses and switching between rules for action consequences (Isoda and Hikosaka 2007). Taken together, the observed decreased ReHo values in the OFC and SMA (particularly the pre-SMA) of patients with migraine without aura in the study by Yu et al. may have been related to deficits in affective pain modulation and affective pain response inhibition.

3.3.2 Gender-Related Differences in Resting-State Networks Dysfunction in Migraine

Migraine is known as gender specific, which is more prevalent in women than men. However, the underlying dysfunctional brain organization accounting for the gender-specific characteristics of migraine is little known. Liu et al. used resting-state fMRI to evaluate resting networks that were conceived as neurocognitive entities incorporating both local and global processes (Liu et al. 2011). Hypothesized differences in the topological properties of these networks were analyzed using a GTA, and functional brain networks were constructed to characterize interregional relationships, small worldness, network resilience, and node centrality in the brains of migraine patients and healthy control subjects. Importantly, networks were constructed using automated anatomically labeled template images (Tzourio-Mazoyer et al. 2002), which divided the whole brain into 90 regions of interest (ROIs). Based on the 90 ROIs as a set of nodes, the mean time series in each ROI were extracted and used to construct a 90×90 matrix of Pearson correlation coefficients for all possible node pair connections. The constructed network was used to calculate interregional connections, and the disruption in the topological properties of these networks was analyzed using a two-way ANOVA performed according to model gender (male vs. female) and disease state (patient vs. control) effects simultaneously. In the results, several pairs of connections were significantly altered in migraine patients with respect to control subjects ($P < 0.05$, false discovery rate corrected). In male migraineurs, connections were significantly increased in the PFC, supramarginal gyrus, amygdala, HIP, IPL, and temporal lobes (Fig. 3.9). The brain regions showing significant increased interregional correlations in

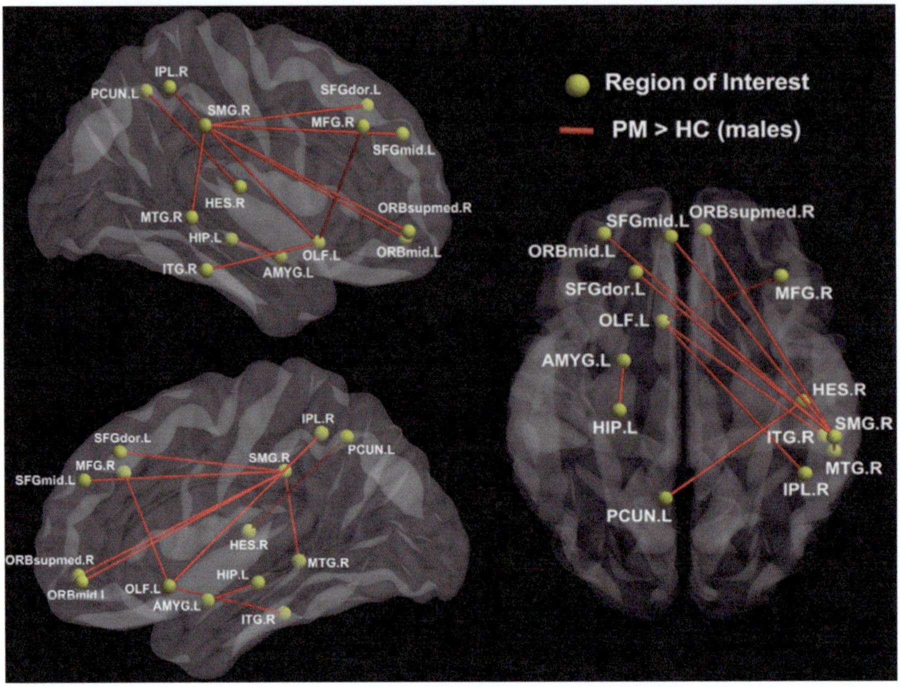

Fig. 3.9 Significant differences in resting-state functional connectivities in male migraineur patients (PM) versus healthy control subjects (HC) (Reprint from Liu et al. 2011). The *red* lines indicated increased intensity in male PMs ($P < 0.05$, corrected). *AMYG*, amygdala; *HES*, Heschl gyrus; *HIP*, hippocampus; *IPL*, inferior parietal lobe; *ITG*, Inferior temporal gyrus; *MFG*, middle frontal gyrus; *MTG*, middle temporal gyrus; *OLF*, Olfactory cortex; *PCUN*, precuneus; *SMG*, Supramarginal gyrus

female migraineurs included the orbital PFC, posterior cingulate gyrus, parahippocampal gyrus, cuneus, putamen, caudate, parietal lobule, temporal lobes, and occipital cortex (Fig. 3.10). No connections were found significantly decreased in migraineurs with respect to control subjects.

Liu et al. found that, compared with matched controls, the interregional correlations of many functional connections were significantly increased, mainly in the primary somatosensory cortex, secondary somatosensory cortex, supramarginal gyrus, PFC, striatum, hippocampus, parahippocampal gyrus, amygdala, occipital cortices, and temporal cortices (Liu et al. 2011). Many of these regions were significantly activated during noxious stimulation in order to mediate the unpleasant-affective dimension of pain and the motivation to escape the stimulus (Treede et al. 1999; Chiapparini et al. 2010; Kang et al. 2010). According to previous studies (May 2009b; Chiapparini et al. 2010), dysfunctional interregional correlations within the pain processing network can be interpreted as a form of brain injury and may thus be secondary to migraine. It was noteworthy that abnormal functional connectivities in migraineurs were skewed between

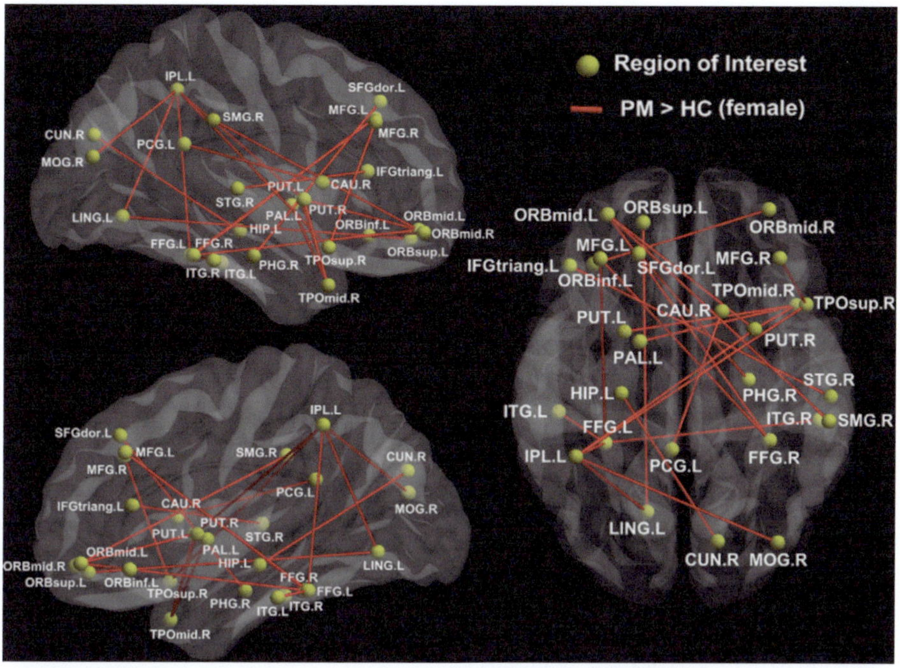

Fig. 3.10 Significant differences in resting-state functional connectivities in female migraineur patients (PM) versus healthy control subjects (HC) (Reprint from Liu et al. 2011). The *red* lines indicated increased intensity in female PMs ($P < 0.05$, corrected). *PreCG* precentral gyrus, *SFGdor* dorsolateral superior frontal gyrus, *ORBinf* orbital inferior frontal gyrus, *ACG* anterior cingulate gyrus, *PHG* parahippocampal gyrus

males and females: in the work by Liu and colleagues, more connection abnormalities were found in the resting networks of female patients. It was reported that migraine was associated with an increased risk of white matter abnormalities in female but not male patients (Zaidat 2004). This may be due to gender differences in brain network organization (Gong et al. 2009, 2011; Tian et al. 2011; Yan et al. 2011). Studies have shown that white matter was more efficiently utilized in women than in men (Gur et al. 1999; Gong et al. 2009). In the previous study employing diffusion tensor imaging tractography, higher overall global and local efficiency was found in the cortical networks of women (Gong et al. 2009). Gur et al. (1999) also found a stronger association between white matter volume and cognitive performance in women than in men (Gur et al. 1999). These differences may provide a basis for the gender-specific characteristics of migraine such as those in the abovementioned results. Specifically, it was possible that the distinct features of female cortical networks were more vulnerable to migraine-related damage and also accounted for the different prevalences of migraine between males and females.

3.4 Mechanisms of Functional Dyspepsia (FD)

FD is a prevalent functional gastrointestinal disorder that has a high worldwide prevalence (Zeng et al. 2011). It was reported that 23.5% of individuals were found to have FD, as indicated in a Chinese population-based epidemiology study. The FD had greatly affected health-related quality of life (QOL) (Talley et al. 2006), and its high economic burden (Moayyedi and Mason 2002) made FD a serious socioeconomic problem.

The pathophysiology of FD remained unclear; theories included gastrointestinal motility abnormalities, visceral hypersensitivity, *Helicobacter pylori* infection, and psychological factors. The symptoms of FD included chronic or recurrent postprandial fullness, early satiation, and epigastric pain or burning thought to originate in the gastroduodenal region in the absence of any underlying organic, systemic, or metabolic disease (Geeraerts and Tack 2008). Although the underlying mechanism of FD was still not completely understood (Zeng et al. 2011), it was found that the disease was related to the abnormal processing of visceral discomfort or pain at the level of the central nervous system (CNS), particularly as related to dysfunction of the brain-gut axis (Van Oudenhove et al. 2004). Using neuroimaging, investigators have confirmed the presence of abnormal brain responses to visceral stimuli as well as during the resting state in patients with FD (Vandenberghe et al. 2007; Van Oudenhove et al. 2010; Zeng et al. 2011).

3.4.1 White Matter Microstructural Changes in Functional Dyspepsia

As indicated in the Rome III criteria (Drossman and Dumitrascu 2006), FD was categorized as: (1) postprandial distress syndrome (PDS), such as meal-related discomfort including postprandial fullness and early satiation, and (2) epigastric pain. Meal-related discomfort and noxious epigastric sensations were inputted to the CNS via distinct afferent pathways (Grundy 2002). Previous study revealed that chronic or recurrent visceral pain was transmitted to the CNS through the spinal afferent pathway (Grundy 2002) and was closely related with brain changes in patients with functional gastrointestinal disorders including irritable bowel syndrome (Blankstein et al. 2010; Seminowicz et al. 2010; Chen et al. 2011) and chronic pancreatitis (Frokjaer et al. 2011). Alternatively, visceral sensations of discomfort were conveyed to the CNS via the vagal afferent pathway (Grundy 2002); moreover, it was unknown whether brain microstructural changes occur in patients with PDS.

To partially address the issue of microstructural alterations in PDS patients, Zhou et al. investigated the white matter (WM) integrity changes in patients with PDS (Zhou et al. 2013). Zhou et al. employed the tract-based spatial statistics method to identify the changes of DTI metrics, including fractional anisotropy (FA), mean diffusivity (MD), axial diffusivity, and radial diffusivity (RD). They also studied the correlations between DTI measures and clinical variables using nonparametric permutation-based tests, and multiple comparisons were corrected using the

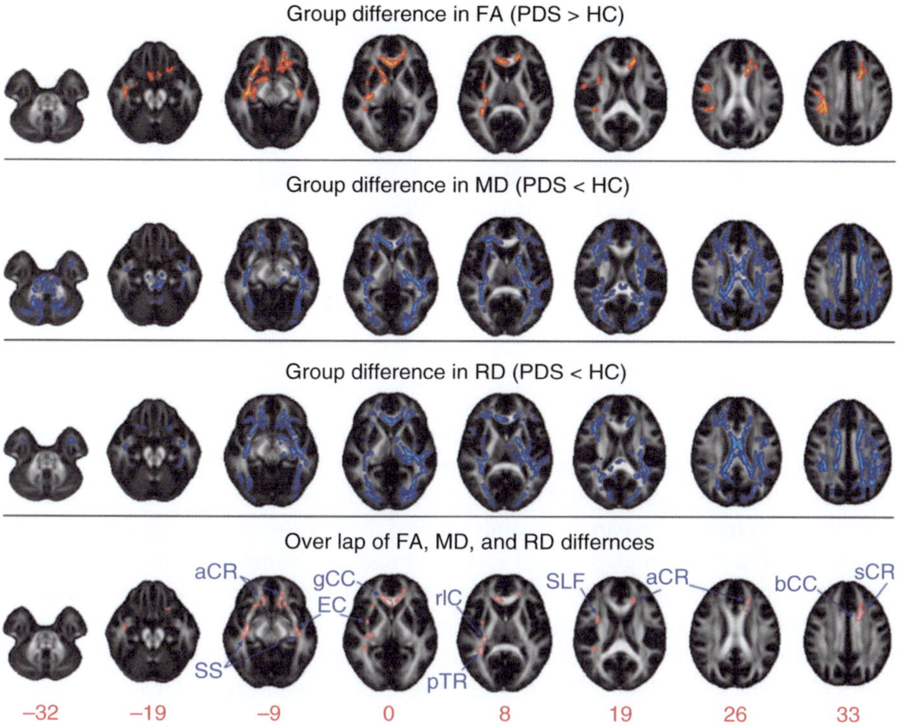

Fig. 3.11 Tract-based spatial statistics findings with the inclusion of age and gender as covariates (Reprint with permission from Zhou et al. 2013)

threshold-free cluster enhancement method. In comparison with the healthy control subjects, increased FA and decreased MD and RD were observed in multiple brain regions among the PDS groups (Zhou et al. 2013). The detailed higher FA values, lower MD, and lower RD values in the PDS were illustrated in Fig. 3.11.

Of note, the WM tracts of increased FA, decreased MD, and RD values were mainly distributed in the WM projection between the frontal lobe and thalamus or between hemispheres. For example, the external capsule contained association fibers such as the inferior fronto-occipital fasciculus, uncinate fasciculus, and superior longitudinal fasciculus. The superior longitudinal fasciculus connected the occipital, parietal, and temporal lobes to the frontal lobe, terminated in the dorsolateral PFC (Jellison et al. 2004). The corona radiata, internal capsule, and posterior thalamic radiate were the projection fiber bundles connecting the cerebral cortex to the thalamus. The corpus callosum interconnected the bilateral homologous brain regions (Jellison et al. 2004) and facilitated interhemispheric communication (Schulte et al. 2005; Whitford et al. 2010). The findings of increased myelination in these tracts might indicate the increased structural connectivity between connected brain regions (Rouw and Scholte 2007), which also represented the disrupted functional connectivity in PDS patients (Greicius et al. 2009; Camchong et al. 2011).

This was supported by the notion that myelin changes alter the conduction efficiency and synchronization of neural signals (Fields 2008; Scholz et al. 2009). In summary, the findings of Zhou and colleagues provided preliminary evidence of WM microstructural changes in patients with PDS. However, given that these changes could be at least partially attributable to a higher level of psychosocial distress in the patient group, additional research was required to determine the direct pertinence of microstructural changes to PDS.

3.4.2 Abnormal Resting-State Brain Activity in Patients with FD

While the pathophysiology of FD remains unclear, a decade of neuroimaging research has demonstrated that FD involves, to some extent, abnormal processing of visceral sensation at the level of the CNS. However, a majority of these studies were performed on irritable bowel syndrome patients, whereas only a few studies were directly conducted on FD patients (Van Oudenhove et al. 2007; Mayer et al. 2009). In addition, most of previous researches mainly studied the CNS responses to painful and/or nonpainful visceral stimulation and identified task- or stimulus-related increases in neural metabolism that were usually small (<5%) relative to resting energy consumption. Spontaneous neural activity can provide more comprehensive information on brain function and has been useful in elucidating the pathogenesis of some disease states (Buckner et al. 2008). Yet, resting-state neuroimaging studies were limited in the context of FD. Zeng et al. compared resting-state brain glycometabolism between FD patients and healthy control subjects using fluorine-18 fluorodeoxyglucose positron emission tomography-computed tomography (PET-CT) and found that FD patients showed higher glycometabolism in the bilateral frontal superior medial gyrus, frontal middle orbital gyrus, ACC, MCC, insula, cerebellum, thalamus, precentral gyrus, postcentral gyrus, middle temporal gyrus, superior temporal gyrus and putamen, right parahippocampal gyrus and claustrum, and left precuneus ($P < 0.001$, family-wise error corrected, minimal cluster size of 50 voxels) (Zeng et al. 2011). The increased glycometabolism was also in the ACC, MCC, anterior insula, thalamus, and cerebellum which were positively correlated with Symptom Index of Dyspepsia score and negatively correlated with Nepean Dyspepsia Index score (Fig. 3.12).

Increased glycometabolism in the anterior cingulate cortex (ACC), insula, thalamus, middle cingulate cortex (MCC), and cerebellum showed significant positive correlations with Symptom Index of Dyspepsia (SID) score and significant negative correlations with the Nepean Dyspepsia Index (NDI) score.

In Zeng's study, areas showing higher glycometabolism in FD patients relative to healthy control subjects were notably main components of the gastric sensation neuromatrix (Van Oudenhove et al. 2007, 2008; Buckner et al. 2008) and involved in the homeostatic afferent network (Mayer et al. 2006), cortical modulatory network, and emotional arousal network. Specifically, the ACC, thalamus, MCC, and insula were essential nodes in the homeostatic afferent network. Increased glycometabolism in these regions might have been related to abnormal homeostatic regulation in FD patients.

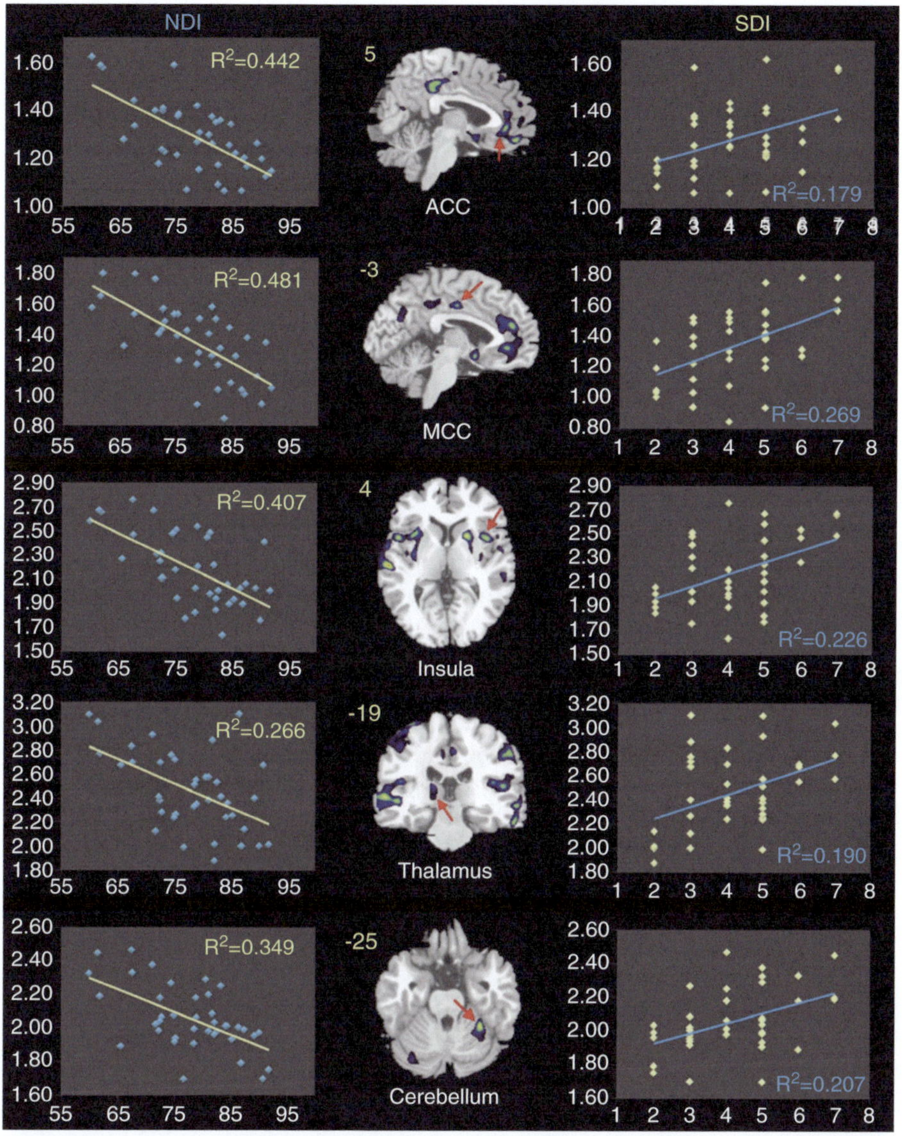

Fig. 3.12 Differences in cerebral glycometabolism between functional dyspepsia (FD) patients and healthy control subjects (Reprint with permission from Zeng et al. 2011)

The PFC was classically included in the cortical modulatory network and played an important role in governing cognitive function. Zeng and colleagues hypothesized that increased activity in the PFC and in other cognitive regions in FD patients may have been due to selectively attending to visceral sensations such as postprandial upper abdominal discomfort and abdominal distension (Zeng et al. 2011).

Finally, the pregenual cingulate cortex, insula, and parahippocampal gyrus were key regions in the emotional arousal network. Although the abovementioned imaging results reported by Zhang and colleagues were obtained after controlling for emotional variables (Riker Sedation-Agitation Scale [SAS] and Zung Self-Rating Depression Scale [SDS] scores), the authors found that the influence of emotional variables on brain glycometabolism was insignificant after comparing controlled and uncontrolled results (not reported in this article). Possible reasons for this observation were as follows: (1) although there were significant differences in SAS and SDS scores between FD patients and healthy control subjects, the anxiety and depression scores of most FD patients were still within the normal range; and (2) most of the key regions showing increased glycometabolism in PD patients, such as the ACC and insula, pertain to the integration cortex and were involved in the processing of visceral and somatic sensory input, emotion, cognition, and behavior. Multiple factors including dyspepsia symptoms and memories of past experiences in addition to cognitive and emotional factors might account for the observation of abnormal cerebral activity in FD patients.

3.4.3 Influence of Acupuncture Treatment on Cerebral Activity in FD Patients

In China and some other Asian countries, acupuncture has been used as a major medical resource for the treatment of gastrointestinal symptoms for several millennia. Nowadays, the acupuncture is also more and more used as an alternative treatment for functional gastrointestinal disorders in the western countries (Takahashi 2006). In the past decade, there have been a lot of clinical and experimental studies which found that the acupuncture was helpful for relieving gastric symptoms such as excessive eructation, abdominal distension, and stomachache by altering gastrointestinal motility (Xu et al. 2006; Yi et al. 2006; Yin and Chen 2010). In addition, acupuncture points on the stomach meridian have been identified as specific effective sites for the treatment of gastric disorders (Xu et al. 2006; Yi et al. 2006). Yet, the exact mechanism of how true acupuncture needling at specific acupoints mediates these therapeutic effects remained unclear.

As abovementioned, Zeng et al. previously demonstrated that altered glycometabolism areas of the homeostatic afferent processing network including the ACC, insula, and thalamus/hypothalamus were related to the severity of FD (Zeng et al. 2011). In subsequent research, this group hypothesized that electroacupuncture therapy might regulate the activity of these key regions and specifically attenuate glycometabolic abnormalities in FD patients (Zeng et al. 2012). A total of 72 FD patients were randomly assigned to receive either electroacupuncture or sham electroacupuncture treatment for 4 weeks, and ten patients in each group were randomly selected to undergo PET-CT. To detect changes in cerebral activity after treatment, differences in cerebral glycometabolism were compared between baseline and post-treatment. Paired t-tests were used to construct statistical parametric maps. The authors found that decreases in cerebral glycometabolism were observed in the

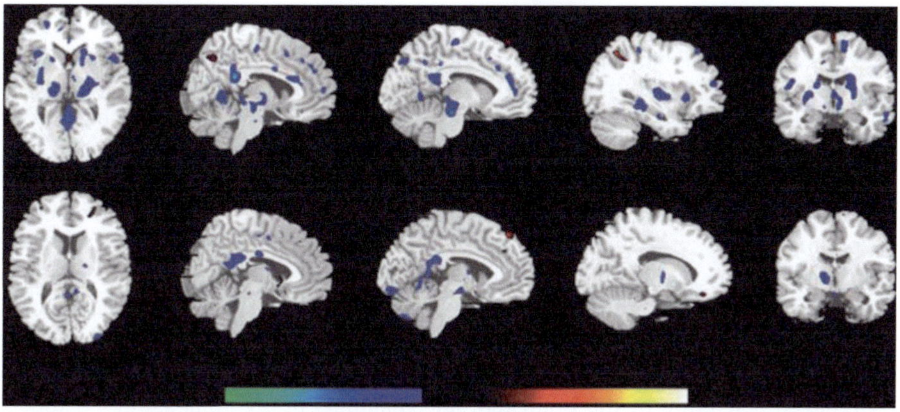

Fig. 3.13 The cerebral glycometabolism of functional dyspepsia (FD) patients changes after treatment (Reprint with permission from Zeng et al. 2012)

acupuncture group after treatment in the bilateral brainstem, cerebellum, ACC, MCC, PCC, and so on. Increases in cerebral glycometabolism were observed in the right postcentral gyrus, bilateral precuneus, and left parietal inferior lobe. In the sham group, both decreased signal and increased signal were observed. The decreased signal was mainly distributed in the bilateral brainstem, thalamus, PCC, left cerebellum, right MCC, lingual gyrus, middle temporal gyrus, middle occipital gyrus, and precuneus. The increased signal was mainly found in the bilateral caudate, left superior medial frontal gyrus, gyrus rectus, and precentral gyrus (Fig. 3.13) (Zeng et al. 2012). Finally, comparing results between the sham and true acupuncture groups, glycometabolism in the bilateral ACC, putamen, thalamus, middle frontal gyrus, middle temporal gyrus, and so on was significantly affected (reduced) by acupuncture in FD patients ($P < 0.001$, uncorrected, minimal cluster size of 20 voxels) (Zeng et al. 2012).

In the work of Zeng et al., both electroacupuncture treatment and sham treatment have shown alterations in cerebral glycometabolism, with commonly responsive areas including the brainstem, thalamus, and regions of the PFC. It was found that the decreased glycometabolism in the brainstem and thalamus was significantly and negatively related to NDI score in the acupuncture group ($P < 0.05$, corrected), whereas this association was nonsignificant in the sham acupuncture group. This might indicate that improvements in QOL might be associated with deactivation of the brainstem and thalamus in PD patients. The brainstem connected the spinal cord/periphery and the highest parts of the brain and also played a role in the functions including visceral regulation, pain sensitivity control, and consciousness. It was known that the physiological status of the gut was directly transmitted to the brainstem to modulate gastric function. The thalamic was crucial for relaying sensation, spatial sense, and motor signals to the cerebral cortex. Previous studies have shown that cerebral glycometabolism was enhanced in the brainstem and thalamus of FD patients relative to healthy subjects (Zeng et al. 2011) and additionally that short-term manual acupuncture treatment can decrease cerebral glycometabolism in the brainstem and thalamus of FD patients (Zeng et al. 2009). In the present study, 4-week electroacupuncture treatment was used to stimulate the somatic afferent nerves. Given that somatic sensory information was projected to various brainstem and thalami nuclei, it can be hypothesized that deactivations in the brainstem and thalamus were a common result of sham acupuncture, manual acupuncture, and electroacupuncture and might not be related to acupuncture point/therapeutic specificity.

In the work by Zeng and colleagues, the acupuncture and sham groups possibly represent manifested similar clinical improvements and cerebral responses. Several recent studies have described the effects of placebo on neural processing. For example, similar to Zeng's findings, both analgesia and placebo effect were accompanied by reduced activation of the brainstem and thalamus in previous studies (Eippert et al. 2009; Qiu et al. 2009). However, it was important to note that some differences in both clinical variables and neuroimaging data between the two groups suggested that the placebo effect does not fully explain the observed effects of acupuncture in Zeng's study. Future studies are required to more carefully separate the effects of placebo from those of acupuncture in the context of FD.

3.5 Summary

As an important complementary and alternative medicine, acupuncture has shown promise for postoperative use and for lessening chemotherapy-induced nausea and vomiting and postoperative dental pain. Furthermore, acupuncture might provide an alternative treatment for drug addiction, asthma, chronic pain, and stroke rehabilitation, though evidence for these indications is minimal and requires additional validation. Acupuncture has been shown to activate different types of afferent nerve fibers, and its effectiveness has been suggested to be dependent on individual symptoms and previous sensitization to acupuncture. Clinical reports further indicate that acupuncture can also modulate the physiological homeostasis to produce treatment effects in patients. Because these observations need further validation, quantitative neuroimaging can provide a useful rationale for the interactions of disease-specific neural correlates and acupuncture-targeted regulatory encoding in the brain. This chapter outlines a series of disease-specific neuroimaging observations in the hopes of facilitating this future research.

References

Apkarian AV, Bushnell MC, Treede RD, et al. Human brain mechanisms of pain perception and regulation in health and disease. Eur J Pain. 2005;9(4):463–84.

Aron AR, Poldrack RA. Cortical and subcortical contributions to stop signal response inhibition: role of the subthalamic nucleus. J Neurosci. 2006;26(9):2424–33.

Balleine BW, Dickinson A. Goal-directed instrumental action: contingency and incentive learning and their cortical substrates. Neuropharmacology. 1998;37(4–5):407–19.

Bechara A, Damasio AR, Damasio H, et al. Insensitivity to future consequences following damage to human prefrontal cortex. Cognition. 1994;50(1–3):7–15.

Blankstein U, Chen J, Diamant NE, et al. Altered brain structure in irritable bowel syndrome: potential contributions of pre-existing and disease-driven factors. Gastroenterology. 2010;138(5):1783–9.

Bonson KR, Grant SJ, Contoreggi CS, et al. Neural systems and cue-induced cocaine craving. Neuropsychopharmacology. 2002;26(3):376–86.

Buckner RL, Andrews-Hanna JR, Schacter DL. The brain's default network: anatomy, function, and relevance to disease. Ann N Y Acad Sci. 2008;1124:1–38.

Buttner A, Mall G, Penning R, et al. The neuropathology of heroin abuse. Forensic Sci Int. 2000;113(1–3):435–42.

Camchong J, MacDonald AW III, Bell C, et al. Altered functional and anatomical connectivity in Schizophrenia. Schizophr Bull. 2011;37(3):640–50.

Caspers S, Geyer S, Schleicher A, et al. The human inferior parietal cortex: cytoarchitectonic parcellation and interindividual variability. NeuroImage. 2006;33(2):430–48.

Chen JY, Blankstein U, Diamant NE, et al. White matter abnormalities in irritable bowel syndrome and relation to individual factors. Brain Res. 2011;1392:121–31.

Chiapparini L, Ferraro S, Grazzi L, et al. Neuroimaging in chronic migraine. Neurol Sci. 2010;31(Suppl 1):S19–22.

Curtis CE, Cole MW, Rao VY, et al. Canceling planned action: an fMRI study of countermanding saccades. Cereb Cortex. 2005;15(9):1281–9.

Drossman DA, Dumitrascu DL. Rome III: new standard for functional gastrointestinal disorders. J Gastrointestin Liver Dis. 2006;15(3):237–41.

Due DL, Huettel SA, Hall WG, et al. Activation in mesolimbic and visuospatial neural circuits elicited by smoking cues: evidence from functional magnetic resonance imaging. Am J Psychiatry. 2002;159(6):954–60.

Eippert F, Bingel U, Schoell ED, et al. Activation of the opioidergic descending pain control system underlies placebo analgesia. Neuron. 2009;63(4):533–43.

Elliott R, Dolan RJ, Frith CD. Dissociable functions in the medial and lateral orbitofrontal cortex: evidence from human neuroimaging studies. Cereb Cortex. 2000;10(3):308–17.

Fields RD. White matter in learning, cognition and psychiatric disorders. Trends Neurosci. 2008;31(7):361–70.

Fox MD, Raichle ME. Spontaneous fluctuations in brain activity observed with functional magnetic resonance imaging. Nat Rev Neurosci. 2007;8(9):700–11.

Fransson P. Spontaneous low-frequency BOLD signal fluctuations: an fMRI investigation of the resting-state default mode of brain function hypothesis. Hum Brain Mapp. 2005;26(1):15–29.

Fransson P, Marrelec G. The precuneus/posterior cingulate cortex plays a pivotal role in the default mode network: evidence from a partial correlation network analysis. NeuroImage. 2008;42(3):1178–84.

Frokjaer JB, Olesen SS, Gram M, et al. Altered brain microstructure assessed by diffusion tensor imaging in patients with chronic pancreatitis. Gut. 2011;60(11):1554–62.

Fu LP, Bi GH, Zou ZT, et al. Impaired response inhibition function in abstinent heroin dependents: an fMRI study. Neurosci Lett. 2008;438(3):322–6.

Garavan H, Pankiewicz J, Bloom A, et al. Cue-induced cocaine craving: neuroanatomical specificity for drug users and drug stimuli. Am J Psychiatry. 2000;157(11):1789–98.

Garrity AG, Pearlson GD, McKiernan K, et al. Aberrant "default mode" functional connectivity in schizophrenia. Am J Psychiatry. 2007;164(3):450–7.

Geeraerts B, Tack J. Functional dyspepsia: past, present, and future. J Gastroenterol. 2008;43(4):251–5.

Goldstein RZ, Volkow ND. Drug addiction and its underlying neurobiological basis: neuroimaging evidence for the involvement of the frontal cortex. Am J Psychiatry. 2002;159(10):1642–52.

Goldstein RZ, Alia-Klein N, Tomasi D, et al. Is decreased prefrontal cortical sensitivity to monetary reward associated with impaired motivation and self-control in cocaine addiction? Am J Psychiatry. 2007;164(1):43–51.

Gong G, Rosa-Neto P, Carbonell F, et al. Age- and gender-related differences in the cortical anatomical network. J Neurosci. 2009;29(50):15684–93.

Gong G, He Y, Evans AC. Brain connectivity: gender makes a difference. Neuroscientist. 2011;17(5):575–91.

Greicius MD, Krasnow B, Reiss AL, et al. Functional connectivity in the resting brain: a network analysis of the default mode hypothesis. Proc Natl Acad Sci U S A. 2003;100(1):253–8.

Greicius MD, Supekar K, Menon V, et al. Resting-state functional connectivity reflects structural connectivity in the default mode network. Cereb Cortex. 2009;19(1):72–8.

Groenewegen HJ, Uylings HB. The prefrontal cortex and the integration of sensory, limbic and autonomic information. Prog Brain Res. 2000;126:3–28.

Grundy D. Neuroanatomy of visceral nociception: vagal and splanchnic afferent. Gut. 2002;51:I2–5.

Gur RC, Turetsky BI, Matsui M, et al. Sex differences in brain gray and white matter in healthy young adults: correlations with cognitive performance. J Neurosci. 1999;19(10):4065–72.

Isoda M, Hikosaka O. Switching from automatic to controlled action by monkey medial frontal cortex. Nat Neurosci. 2007;10(2):240–8.

Jellison BJ, Field AS, Medow J, et al. Diffusion tensor imaging of cerebral white matter: a pictorial review of physics, fiber tract anatomy, and tumor imaging patterns. AJNR Am J Neuroradiol. 2004;25(3):356–69.

Kang DH, Son JH, Kim YC. Neuroimaging studies of chronic pain. The Korean J Pain. 2010;23(3):159–65.

Kaufman JN, Ross TJ, Stein EA, et al. Cingulate hypoactivity in cocaine users during a GO-NOGO task as revealed by event-related functional magnetic resonance imaging. J Neurosci. 2003;23(21):7839–43.

Krawczyk DC. Contributions of the prefrontal cortex to the neural basis of human decision making. Neurosci Biobehav Rev. 2002;26(6):631–64.

Kupers RC, Gybels JM, Gjedde A. Positron emission tomography study of a chronic pain patient successfully treated with somatosensory thalamic stimulation. Pain. 2000;87(3):295–302.

Lee TM, Pau CW. Impulse control differences between abstinent heroin users and matched controls. Brain Inj. 2002;16(10):885–9.

Lee TM, Zhou WH, Luo XJ, et al. Neural activity associated with cognitive regulation in heroin users: a fMRI study. Neurosci Lett. 2005;382(3):211–6.

Li CS, Sinha R. Inhibitory control and emotional stress regulation: neuroimaging evidence for frontal-limbic dysfunction in psycho-stimulant addiction. Neurosci Biobehav Rev. 2008;32(3):581–97.

Li CS, Huang C, Constable RT, et al. Imaging response inhibition in a stop-signal task: neural correlates independent of signal monitoring and post-response processing. J Neurosci. 2006;26(1):186–92.

Lieberman MD, Jarcho JM, Berman S, et al. The neural correlates of placebo effects: a disruption account. NeuroImage. 2004;22(1):447–55.

Liu J, Liang J, Qin W, et al. Dysfunctional connectivity patterns in chronic heroin users: an fMRI study. Neurosci Lett. 2009;460(1):72–7.

Liu J, Qin W, Nan J, et al. Gender-related differences in the dysfunctional resting networks of migraine suffers. PLoS One. 2011;6(11):e27049.

Lyoo IK, Streeter CC, Ahn KH, et al. White matter hyperintensities in subjects with cocaine and opiate dependence and healthy comparison subjects. Psychiatry Res. 2004;131(2):135–45.

Lyoo IK, Pollack MH, Silveri MM, et al. Prefrontal and temporal gray matter density decreases in opiate dependence. Psychopharmacology. 2006;184(2):139–44.

Ma N, Liu Y, Li N, et al. Addiction related alteration in resting-state brain connectivity. NeuroImage. 2010;49(1):738–44.

MacDonald AW, Cohen JD, Stenger VA, et al. Dissociating the role of the dorsolateral prefrontal and anterior cingulate cortex in cognitive control. Science. 2000;288(5472):1835–8.

May A. Morphing voxels: the hype around structural imaging of headache patients. Brain. 2009a;132:1419–25.

May A. New insights into headache: an update on functional and structural imaging findings. Nat Rev Neurol. 2009b;5(4):199–209.
Mayer EA, Naliboff BD, Craig AD. Neuroimaging of the brain-gut axis: from basic understanding to treatment of functional G1 disorders. Gastroenterology. 2006;131(6):1925–42.
Mayer EA, Aziz Q, Coen S, et al. Brain imaging approaches to the study of functional GI disorders: a Rome working team report. Neurogastroenterol Motil. 2009;21(6):579–96.
Mechias ML, Etkin A, Kalisch R. A meta-analysis of instructed fear studies: implications for conscious appraisal of threat. NeuroImage. 2010;49(2):1760–8.
Moayyedi P, Mason J. Clinical and economic consequences of dyspepsia in the community. Gut. 2002;50:10–2.
Monterosso JR, Aron AR, Cordova X, et al. Deficits in response inhibition associated with chronic methamphetamine abuse. Drug Alcohol Depend. 2005;79(2):273–7.
Nachev P, Rees G, Parton A, et al. Volition and conflict in human medial frontal cortex. Curr Biol. 2005;15(2):122–8.
Park MS, Sohn JH, Suk JA, et al. Brain substrates of craving to alcohol cues in subjects with alcohol use disorder. Alcohol Alcohol. 2007;42(5):417–22.
Petrovic P, Kalso E, Petersson KM, et al. Placebo and opioid analgesia: imaging a shared neuronal network. Science. 2002;295(5560):1737–40.
Phillips ML, Drevets WC, Rauch SL, et al. Neurobiology of emotion perception I: the neural basis of normal emotion perception. Biol Psychiatry. 2003;54(5):504–14.
Picard N, Strick PL. Motor areas of the medial wall: a review of their location and functional activation. Cereb Cortex. 1996;6(3):342–53.
Ploghaus A, Tracey I, Gati JS, et al. Dissociating pain from its anticipation in the human brain. Science. 1999;284(5422):1979–81.
Qiu YH, XY W, Xu H, et al. Neuroimaging study of placebo analgesia in humans. Neurosci Bull. 2009;25(5):277–82.
Rouw R, Scholte HS. Increased structural connectivity in grapheme-color synesthesia. Nat Neurosci. 2007;10(6):792–7.
Roy M, Piche M, Chen JI, et al. Cerebral and spinal modulation of pain by emotions. Proc Natl Acad Sci U S A. 2009;106(49):20900–5.
Rushworth MF, Walton ME, Kennerley SW, et al. Action sets and decisions in the medial frontal cortex. Trends Cogn Sci. 2004;8(9):410–7.
Scholz J, Klein MC, Behrens TE, et al. Training induces changes in white-matter architecture. Nat Neurosci. 2009;12(11):1370–1.
Schulte T, Sullivan EV, Muller-Oehring EM, et al. Corpus callosal microstructural integrity influences interhemispheric processing: a diffusion tensor imaging study. Cereb Cortex. 2005;15(9):1384–92.
Schwedt TJ, Dodick DW. Advanced neuroimaging of migraine. Lancet Neurol. 2009;8(6):560–8.
Seminowicz DA, Labus JS, Bueller JA, et al. Regional gray matter density changes in brains of patients with irritable bowel syndrome. Gastroenterology. 2010;139(1):48–57.
Shackman AJ, Salomons TV, Slagter HA, et al. The integration of negative affect, pain and cognitive control in the cingulate cortex. Nat Rev Neurosci. 2011;12(3):154–67.
Shalev U, Grimm JW, Shaham Y. Neurobiology of relapse to heroin and cocaine seeking: a review. Pharmacol Rev. 2002;54(1):1–42.
Sinha R. How does stress increase risk of drug abuse and relapse? Psychopharmacology. 2001;158(4):343–59.
Takahashi T. Acupuncture for functional gastrointestinal disorders. J Gastroenterol. 2006;41(5):408–17.
Talley NJ, Locke GR, Lahr BD, et al. Functional dyspepsia, delayed gastric emptying, and impaired quality of life. Gut. 2006;55(7):933–9.
Terwindt GM, Ferrari MD, Tijhuis M, et al. The impact of migraine on quality of life in the general population: the GEM study. Neurology. 2000;55(5):624–9.
Tian L, Wang J, Yan C, et al. Hemisphere- and gender-related differences in small-world brain networks: a resting-state functional MRI study. NeuroImage. 2011;54(1):191–202.

Tietjen GE. Stroke and migraine linked by silent lesions. Lancet Neurol. 2004;3(5):267.

Treede RD, Kenshalo DR, Gracely RH, et al. The cortical representation of pain. Pain. 1999;79(2–3):105–11.

Tzourio-Mazoyer N, Landeau B, Papathanassiou D, et al. Automated anatomical labeling of activations in SPM using a macroscopic anatomical parcellation of the MNI MRI single-subject brain. NeuroImage. 2002;15(1):273–89.

Van Oudenhove L, Demyttenaere K, Tack J, et al. Central nervous system involvement in functional gastrointestinal disorders. Best Pract Res Clin Gastroenterol. 2004;18(4):663–80.

Van Oudenhove L, Coen SJ, Aziz Q. Functional brain imaging of gastrointestinal sensation in health and disease. World J Gastroenterol. 2007;13(25):3438–45.

Van Oudenhove L, Dupont P, Vandenberghe J, et al. The role of somatosensory cortical regions in the processing of painful gastric fundic distension: an update of brain imaging findings. Neurogastroenterol Motil. 2008;20(5):479–87.

Van Oudenhove L, Vandenberghe J, Dupont P, et al. Regional brain activity in functional dyspepsia: a H(2)(15)O-PET study on the role of gastric sensitivity and abuse history. Gastroenterology. 2010;139(1):36–47.

Vandenberghe J, Dupont P, Van Oudenhove L, et al. Regional cerebral blood flow during gastric balloon distention in functional dyspepsia. Gastroenterology. 2007;132(5):1684–93.

Vanderhasselt MA, De Raedt R, Baeken C. Dorsolateral prefrontal cortex and Stroop performance: tackling the lateralization. Psychon Bull Rev. 2009;16(3):609–12.

Vincent M, Pedra E, Mourao-Miranda J, et al. Enhanced interictal responsiveness of the migraineous visual cortex to incongruent bar stimulation: a functional MRI visual activation study. Cephalalgia. 2003;23(9):860–8.

Vogt BA. Pain and emotion interactions in subregions of the cingulate gyrus. Nat Rev Neurosci. 2005;6(7):533–44.

Volkow ND, Fowler JS, Wang GJ. The addicted human brain: insights from imaging studies. J Clin Invest. 2003;111(10):1444–51.

Wager TD, Rilling JK, Smith EE, et al. Placebo-induced changes in fMRI in the anticipation and experience of pain. Science. 2004;303(5661):1162–7.

Wallis JD, Miller EK. Neuronal activity in primate dorsolateral and orbital prefrontal cortex during performance of a reward preference task. Eur J Neurosci. 2003;18(7):2069–81.

Wang L, Zang Y, He Y, et al. Changes in hippocampal connectivity in the early stages of Alzheimer's disease: evidence from resting state fMRI. NeuroImage. 2006;31(2):496–504.

Whitford TJ, Kubicki M, Schneiderman JS, et al. Corpus callosum abnormalities and their association with psychotic symptoms in patients with schizophrenia. Biol Psychiatry. 2010;68(1):70–7.

Wiech K, Ploner M, Tracey I. Neurocognitive aspects of pain perception. Trends Cogn Sci. 2008;12(8):306–13.

Wilson SJ, Sayette MA, Fiez JA. Prefrontal responses to drug cues: a neurocognitive analysis. Nat Neurosci. 2004;7(3):211–4.

Xiao ZW, Lee T, Zhang JX, et al. Thirsty heroin addicts show different fMRI activations when exposed to water-related and drug-related cues. Drug Alcohol Depend. 2006;83(2):157–62.

Xu S, Hou X, Zha H, et al. Electroacupuncture accelerates solid gastric emptying and improves dyspeptic symptoms in patients with functional dyspepsia. Dig Dis Sci. 2006;51(12):2154–9.

Yan C, Gong G, Wang J, et al. Sex- and brain size-related small-world structural cortical networks in young adults: a DTI tractography study. Cereb Cortex. 2011;21(2):449–58.

Yi SX, Yang RD, Yan J, et al. Effect of electro-acupuncture at Foot-Yangming Meridian on somatostatin and expression of somatostatin receptor genes in rabbits with gastric ulcer. World J Gastroenterol. 2006;12(11):1761–5.

Yin J, Chen JD. Gastrointestinal motility disorders and acupuncture. Auton Neurosci. 2010;157(1–2):31–7.

Yu D, Yuan K, Zhao L, et al. Regional homogeneity abnormalities in patients with interictal migraine without aura: a resting-state study. NMR Biomed. 2012;25(5):806–12.

Yuan Y, Zhu Z, Shi J, et al. Gray matter density negatively correlates with duration of heroin use in young lifetime heroin-dependent individuals. Brain Cogn. 2009;71(3):223–8.

Yuan K, Qin W, Dong M, et al. Combining spatial and temporal information to explore resting-state networks changes in abstinent heroin-dependent individuals. Neurosci Lett. 2010a;475(1):20–4.

Yuan K, Qin W, Dong M, et al. Gray matter deficits and resting-state abnormalities in abstinent heroin-dependent individuals. Neurosci Lett. 2010b;482(2):101–5.

Yuan K, Qin W, Liu J, et al. Altered small-world brain functional networks and duration of heroin use in male abstinent heroin-dependent individuals. Neurosci Lett. 2010c;477(1):37–42.

Yuan K, Qin W, Wang G, et al. Microstructure abnormalities in adolescents with internet addiction disorder. PLoS One. 2011;6(6):e20708.

Zaidat OO. Migraine as a risk factor for subclinical brain lesions. JAMA. 2004;291(17):2072.

Zeng F, Song WZ, Liu XG, et al. Brain areas involved in acupuncture treatment on functional dyspepsia patients: a PET-CT study. Neurosci Lett. 2009;456(1):6–10.

Zeng F, Qin W, Liang F, et al. Abnormal resting brain activity in patients with functional dyspepsia is related to symptom severity. Gastroenterology. 2011;141(2):499–506.

Zeng F, Qin W, Ma T, et al. Influence of acupuncture treatment on cerebral activity in functional dyspepsia patients and its relationship with efficacy. Am J Gastroenterol. 2012;107(8):1236–47.

Zhou Y, Lin FC, YS D, et al. Gray matter abnormalities in internet addiction: a voxel-based morphometry study. Eur J Radiol. 2011;79(1):92–5.

Zhou G, Qin W, Zeng F, et al. White-matter microstructural changes in functional dyspepsia: a diffusion tensor imaging study. Am J Gastroenterol. 2013;108(2):260–9.

Findings of Acupuncture Mechanisms Using EEG and MEG

4

Wei Qin, Lijun Bai, Lingmin Jin, and Jie Tian

4.1 Introduction

Multimodality neuroimaging techniques provide more information about how acupuncture works. EEG and MEG have excellent temporal resolution which may make up the lack of MRI in temporal resolution. We will review recent acupuncture studies using EEG/MEG in this chapter.

In addition to modalities such as functional magnetic resonance imaging (MRI), other noninvasive imaging techniques such as electroencephalography (EEG) and magnetoencephalography (MEG) have been applied to investigate the therapeutic effects of acupuncture. EEG allows the recording of spontaneous cerebral electrical activity over time via electrodes positioned on the scalp surface; MEG is a functional neuroimaging technique that maps brain activity by measuring magnetic fields generated by electrical currents occurring naturally in the brain. Both EEG and MEG have very high temporal resolutions with the ability to resolve time scales on the order of milliseconds. Both of these measurements are painless and generally very safe. This chapter will review the principles of EEG and MEG as well as their use in the study of acupuncture.

W. Qin • L. Jin
School of Life Sciences and Technology, Xidian University, Xi'an, China

L. Bai
The Key Laboratory of Biomedical Information Engineering, Ministry of Education, Department of Biomedical Engineering, School of Life Science and Technology, Xi'an Jiaotong University, Xi'an, China

J. Tian (✉)
CAS Key Laboratory of Molecular Imaging, Institute of Automation, Beijing, China
e-mail: jie.tian@ia.ac.cn

© Springer Nature Singapore Pte Ltd. 2018

J. Tian (ed.), *Multi-Modality Neuroimaging Study on Neurobiological Mechanisms of Acupuncture*, DOI 10.1007/978-981-10-4914-9_4

4.2 Principles of Electroencephalography (EEG)

The human brain is the most complexly organized biological structure known to man. There are at least 10^{10} neurons in the outermost layer of the brain (the cerebral cortex), and these cells are the active units in a vast signaling network that includes more than 10^{14} interconnections. The brain consists of two hemispheres separated by the longitudinal fissure. The left and right hemispheres are further divided into lobes by two deep grooves. Accordingly, there are four lobes in each half of the cortex: the frontal, parietal, temporal, and occipital lobes. Techniques such as electroencephalography (EEG) and magnetoencephalography (MEG) have been used to functionally map most regions of cortex. In this chapter, we will review information about the effects of acupuncture in the brain garnered from EEG and MEG studies.

EEG is a relatively young technique. In 1875, Richard Caton was the first to discover the existence of electrical currents in the brains of rabbits and monkeys using a device called Thomson's mirror galvanometer (Caton 1875). In 1924, Hans Berger, considered the father of modern EEG, recorded the first human EEG using a string galvanometer and first used the word "electroencephalogram" to describe the observed electric potentials (Haas 2003). Later in 1934, Adrian and Matthews published a paper verifying the concept of "human brain waves" and identified regular oscillations around 10–12 Hz that were termed "alpha rhythm." At present, EEG can be performed invasively and noninvasively using fully computerized systems and has facilitated the rapid development of experimental and clinical diagnostic and therapeutic approaches for a vast number of neurological and physiological conditions.

4.2.1 EEG Signal Generation

EEG signal is a measurement of current that is generated from the synaptic excitation of neuronal dendrites in the cerebral cortex. Differences in electrical potential result from the summation of postsynaptic graded potentials that create electrical dipoles between the cell soma (neuronal cell body) and apical dendrites (neuronal branches). Accordingly, brain electrical current is primarily generated by the movement of Na^+, K^+, Ca^{2+}, and Cl^- ions across neuronal membranes, governed by membrane potentials and the function of active ion pumps (Atwood and MacKay 1989). Of course, the detailed microscopic picture is more sophisticated, including different types of synapses and a variety of neurotransmitters.

4.2.2 EEG Recording and Measurement

Traditionally, EEGs were recorded using electromechanical chart recorders. More recent EEG systems are digital, consisting of an electrode cap, amplifier(s) and filter(s), an analog-to-digital converter, and a recording device (Teplan 2002). It is important to note that only large populations of active neurons can generate electrical activity that is recordable on the scalp surface, considering that current must penetrate the brain, skull, scalp, and several other thin layers of tissue. Therefore, after cap electrodes detect microvolt signals from the scalp surface, amplifiers bring these signals into a range where they can be accurately digitalized, converters convert analog signals into digital form, and a personal computer (or other relevant device) stores and displays obtained data. Commonly used scalp electrodes are Ag-AgCl disks, 1–3 mm in diameter, with long flexible leads that can be connected to an amplifier. The space between the electrode and the skin of the scalp is typically filled with a conductive paste to facilitate adhesion and recording. Electrode positions most commonly adopt the 10–20 electrode placement system (Jasper 1958); this system is a standardized electrode designation and physical placement pattern on the scalp. The head is divided into proportional distances from prominent skull landmarks (i.e., the nasion, preauricular points, and inion) to provide adequate coverage of all regions of the brain. The 10–20 label designates the percent proportional distance between the ears and nose where electrodes are placed. Electrode placements are labeled according to adjacent brain areas: F (frontal), C (central), T (temporal), P (posterior), and O (occipital) (Fig. 4.1) (Oostenveld and Praamstra 2001). The

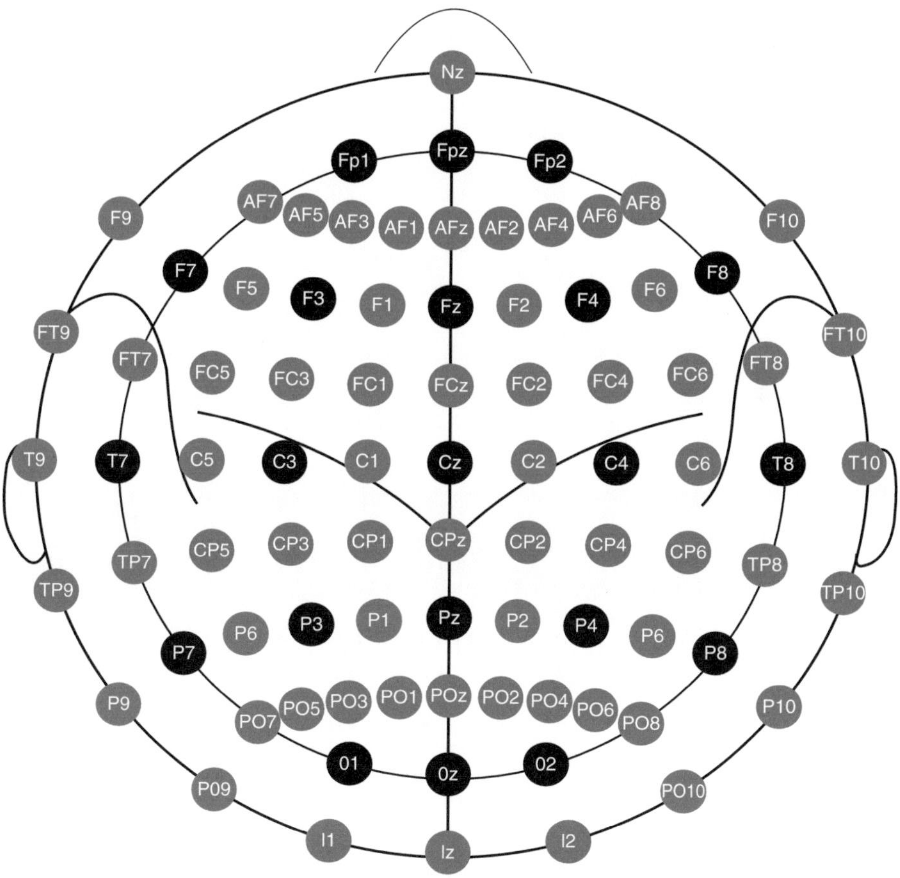

Fig. 4.1 Electrode positions and labels according to the 10–20 electrode placement system. *Black* circles indicate positions of the original 10–20 system, *gray* circles indicate additional positions introduced in the 10–10 extension (Reprint with permission from Oostenveld and Praamstra 2001)

letters are accompanied by odd numbers on the left side of the head and even numbers on the right side of the head (where left and right are considered from the subject's point of view).

4.2.3 EEG Rhythms

There are four basic brain waves distinguished on EEG according to their frequency ranges: delta (0.5–4 Hz), theta (4–7.5 Hz), alpha (8–13 Hz), and beta (14–30 Hz). Delta waves are primarily associated with deep sleep but may be present in the waking state. Theta waves appear as slips of consciousness toward drowsiness and have been associated with access to unconscious material, creative inspiration, and deep meditation. Alpha waves are usually found over the occipital region of the brain. Figure 4.2 shows how the wavelength and alpha frequency were calculated (Johannisson 2016). Most subjects produce some alpha waves when their eyes are closed, and these waves are dampened or eliminated by opening the eyes, hearing unfamiliar sounds, anxiety, or mental concentration or attention. Lastly, beta waves are chiefly found over the frontal and central regions and are characterized by low amplitudes.

In addition to the abovementioned classical waveforms, other brain waveforms have been reported (Iber et al. 2007):

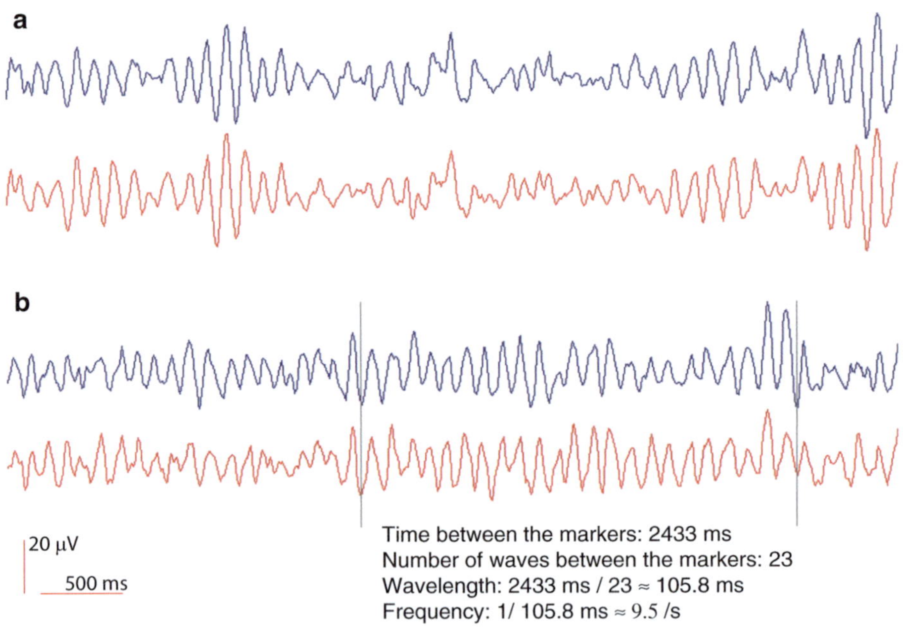

Fig. 4.2 Alpha waves. (**a**) Short sequences of alpha waves. (**b**) An example of a sequence used in the present study. *Blue* tracings are from AFz-TP9 and *red* tracings are from AFz-TP10 (Reprint from Johannisson 2016)

(a) K-complexes are well-delineated negative sharp waves that are immediately followed by a positive component, usually lasting >0.5 s. K-complexes are clearly distinguishable from background EEG noise and are typically maximal in amplitude when recorded using frontal derivations.
(b) Vertex sharp waves are sharply contoured waves with durations <0.5 s. These waves are clearly distinguishable from background activity and are maximal in amplitude over the central region.
(c) Sleep spindles (also called sigma activity) occur within the 11–15 Hz frequency range and are associated with learning, memory, and intelligence.
(d) Slow-wave activity describes waves of 0.5–2 Hz in frequency that have a peak-to-peak amplitude >75 μV, usually measured over frontal regions.
(e) Sawtooth waves are trains of sharply contoured or triangular (often serrated) 2–6 Hz waves that show maximal amplitude over central cranial regions and often, but not always, precede a burst of rapid eye movement (REM).

4.2.4 EEG Applications

Given the wealth of knowledge provided by EEG, it is no surprise that this method has paved the way for the diagnosis and treatment of many neurological disorders and abnormalities in the human body. EEG signals from humans and animals have been used for the investigation of the following clinical problems to date (Bickford 1987):

(a) Monitoring alertness, coma, and brain death
(b) Locating areas of damage following head injury, stroke, and tumor
(c) Testing afferent pathways (using evoked potentials)
(d) Monitoring cognitive engagement (alpha rhythm)
(e) Producing biofeedback situations
(f) Controlling depth of anesthesia (servo anesthesia)
(g) Investigating epilepsy and locating seizure origin
(h) Testing pro-convulsive or anticonvulsive drug effects
(i) Assisting the experimental cortical excision of epileptic foci
(j) Monitoring brain development
(k) Investigating sleep disorder pathophysiology
(l) Investigating mental disorders
(m) Providing a hybrid data recording system together with other imaging modalities

4.3 Applications of EEG in Acupuncture Research

EEG has long been used to understand the neurobiological basis of acupuncture and its effects (Chen and Huang 1984; Chongcheng et al. 1985). We will introduce these animal and human studies separately.

4.3.1 EEG Studies of Acupuncture in Animals

Various animal models have been employed to study the effects of acupuncture in a controlled setting. In a basic research study, He and colleagues evaluated the influence of the duration of interstitial laser acupuncture therapy on brain activity in naïve animals using EEG and HRV. Six rats underwent 10, 20, or 30 min of interstitial laser acupuncture at PC6 in a randomized order with a 30-min break between each condition. The periods of 10 min before, during, and 10 min after laser stimulation were recorded by EEG and HRV in all three conditions (10-, 20-, and 30-min laser acupuncture duration). Whereas HR was significantly altered after the 20-min red laser stimulation, neither the LF/HF ratio of HRV nor the integrated EEG showed any significant between-condition differences (He et al. 2013a). In a preclinical study, the effect of gold wire implants at specific acupoints on uncontrolled idiopathic epileptic seizures was evaluated in canines (Goiz-Marquez et al. 2009). Fifteen dogs with a positive diagnosis were enrolled in the study, and EEG recording was performed before and 15 weeks after the treatment protocol. Relative frequency power, intrahemispheric coherence available from EEG data, number of seizures, and seizure severity were compared before and after treatment using a Wilcoxon signed-rank test. No significant statistical differences were observed in relative power or intrahemispheric coherence; however, there was a significant mean reduction in seizure frequency and seizure severity after treatment. This study suggested that the effects of acupuncture on clinical presentation might not conform with characteristics on EEG.

Another study evaluated the effects of acupuncture on EEG spectral edge frequency (SEF) 95 in dogs sedated with butorphanol (Kim et al. 2006). SEF 95 values were significantly reduced during acupuncture at GV20 or at the EX-HN3 (Yintang) point and returned to the baseline values after acupuncture release. Ramsay sedation score (RSS) values also confirmed an acceptable level of sedation level during acupuncture. It was concluded that acupuncture application at GV20 or the EX-HN3 point used in combination with butorphanol sedation would be a valuable complementary method for inducing and maintaining sedation in dogs (Kim and Nam 2006).

By recording EEG signals in rats, it has found that EA stimulation of Feng-Chi acupoints is beneficial in suppressing focal epilepsy and treating epilepsy-induced sleep disruptions (Yi et al. 2015) (Fig. 4.3). The mechanism of EA in this context, however, is still unclear. One study investigated the effects of Anmian (extra) acupoint EA stimulation on sleep organization and the caudal nucleus tractus solitarius (NTS) using EEG in rats (Yi et al. 2004). One-time EA stimulation 25 min prior to the onset of the dark period enhanced REM sleep. Furthermore, the effects of EA on sleep were precluded by electrical lesion of the bilateral caudal NTS. However, EA stimulation did not alter slow-wave activity during slow-wave sleep, despite the fact that slow-wave activity was reduced after caudal NTS lesion. These results suggested that the caudal NTS might play a role in the effects of EA on sleep.

Panels a, b, c, and d respectively depict the EEG signals recorded from the naïve rats, the pilocarpine group, the PFS (pyrogen-free saline) + EA + pilocarpine

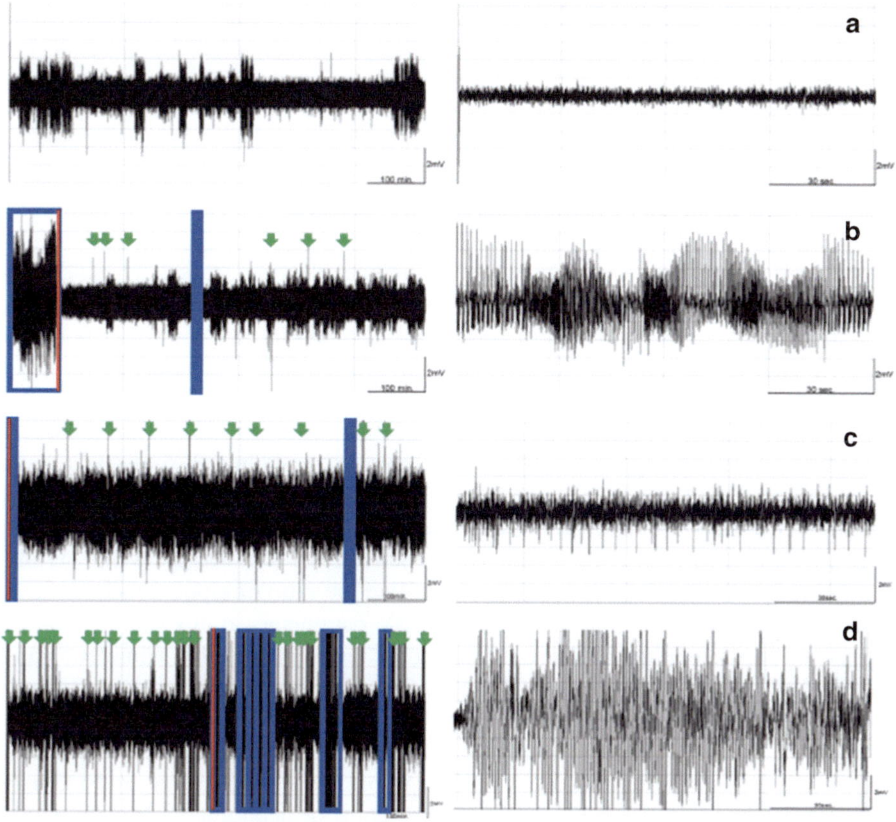

Fig. 4.3 The effect of 10-Hz EA stimulation of bilateral Feng-Chi acupoints and naloxone on epileptic activities (Reprint from Yi et al. 2015)

group, and the naloxone + EA + pilocarpine group, beginning from the dark onset of the dark period. Pilocarpine was administered at time 0 in the left panels of b, c, and d. The blue boxes represent the epileptiform EEGs. Red lines indicate the extracted time points for the expanded time-scale figures in the right panels. Green arrowheads are the artifacts. The larger amplitudes, with EEG signals less than 2 mV that appeared in panels a, were delta waves, which represent the state of slow-wave sleep.

Intravenous (i.v.) laser blood irradiation using a one-way catheter (Gamaleia et al. 1988; Korochkin et al. 1988) and percutaneous interstitial (i.st.) laser therapy using a sterile catheter permit the penetration of laser light into deeper tissues for the treatment of herniated disks or spinal stenosis (Weber 2011). Intravenous (i.v.) laser blood irradiation, interstitial (i.st.) laser acupuncture, and EA were compared using EEG and HRV and were investigated in ten anesthetized male Sprague-Dawley rats. HR was significantly decreased during i.st. laser acupuncture stimulation of Neiguan, while total HRV was nonsignificantly increased during i.v. and i.st.

laser stimulation. The LF/HF ratio only showed significant changes during i.v. laser blood irradiation. Integrated cortical EEG showed insignificant decreases during EA and i.v. laser blood irradiation. Further studies concerning the dose-dependent nature of these effects are in progress (He et al. 2013b).

4.3.2 EEG Studies of Acupuncture in Humans

Studies of healthy volunteers. A number of acupoints had been studied by using EEG to evaluate the specific changes in spontaneous electrical activity in the brain. For example, one study investigated the effects of acupressure at the Extra 1 point on EEG spectral entropy values and heart rate variability (HRV). Compared with sham control, acupressure significantly reduced EEG spectral entropy and decreased the low-frequency/high-frequency (LF/HF) ratio of HRV (Arai et al. 2011). Physiological responses to electroacupuncture (EA) stimulation of acupoints PC5 and PC6 have also been evaluated using EEG and HRV; EA stimulation of these points increased the number of low-frequency waves in all lobes and additionally increased the mean R-R interval (Kim et al. 2009). Manual acupuncture at LI4 was shown to significantly increase the alpha-1 frequency and shifted the ratio of alpha-1/theta to favor alpha-1 at all electrodes (Juel et al. 2016). HRV parameters in this study showed a significant increase in the LF/HF ratio during the first minute of LI4 stimulation and followed by a decrease thereafter. These studies suggest that various acupoint locations and stimulation methods might lead to alterations in EEG and HRV signal.

Distinct analysis methods have been employed in the study of acupuncture. A wavelet-limited penetrable visibility graph approach was used to analyze EEG data from 15 healthy subjects undergoing acupuncture at acupoint ST36. The study found that acupuncture influenced the complexity of EEG sub-bands in different ways and led to higher efficiency and stronger small-world properties of functional brain networks compared with the pre-acupuncture control state (Pei et al. 2014). Another study used an order recurrence quantification analysis combined with discrete wavelet transforms to analyze the dynamic characteristics of different EEG rhythms during ST36 stimulation. Stimulation decreased the complexity of the delta rhythm, increased that of the alpha rhythm, and had no obvious effects on the beta, theta, and gamma rhythms relative to the pre-acupuncture state (Yi et al. 2013).

Magnetic acupuncture is a painless stimulation method and has been recently reported as an effective modality in clinical practice (Colbert et al. 2008). The effects of magnetic stimulation at acupoint HT7 were evaluated by examining event-related potentials (ERPs) on EEG. Colbert and colleagues identified an obvious P150 component in response to magnetic acupuncture using the dipole model. Acupuncture at HT7 was found to evoke stronger activity in the somatosensory cortex than sham stimulation and sham acupoint stimulation (Geng and Zhang 2012). Magnetic LI4 stimulation was also investigated using EEG; a peak potential was recorded at frontal midline (FCZ) electrode sites at about 140–170 ms (likely to be P150) after acupoint stimulation but not non-acupoint stimulation (Yu et al. 2009).

Another study explored the differential effects of acupressure, acupuncture, and laser acupuncture on EEG bispectral index, spectral edge frequency, and verbal sedation score using the acupoint EX-HN3 and a sham point. Bispectral index and spectral edge frequency values both significantly decreased during acupressure stimulation at EX-HN3, and all three interventions significantly reduced verbal sedation score (Litscher 2004).

The effects of laser acupuncture, manual acupuncture, and light stimulation on cerebral blood flow were investigated in 15 healthy volunteers using noninvasive transcranial Doppler sonography and the bispectral index of EEG (Litscher et al. 2000). Light stimulation significantly increased blood flow velocity in the posterior cerebral artery, while a similar but less pronounced effect was seen after manual and laser acupuncture at vision-related acupoints. Furthermore, significant increases in the amplitudes of 40-Hz cerebral oscillations were noted during both laser and manual acupuncture.

The effects of acupuncture at PC6 have also been assessed. Chang et al. reported an increase in the amplitude and power of the alpha band during manual PC6 acupuncture compared to baseline data (Chang et al. 2009). Meanwhile, frequency peaks in the alpha bands of 12 channels were all synchronized with a much smaller standard deviation compared with the baseline data, and these phenomena persisted for at least 10 min after the cessation of stimulation. Kim and his colleagues found the similar results that the power of the frequency bands including alpha-wave, beta-wave, theta-wave, and delta-wave all increased considerably after acupuncture stimulation at PC6 (Kim et al. 2008).

The effects of high- (100 Hz) and low-frequency (2 Hz) transcutaneous electrical nerve stimulation (TENS) at LI4 were compared for the delta, theta, alpha-1, alpha-2, beta, and gamma bands using 124-channel EEG (Chen et al. 2006). The absolute EEG powers (muv2) at focal maxima across three stages (baseline, stimulation, and post-stimulation) were examined by using two-way (condition, stage) repeated measures ANOVA. Theta power activity was significantly decreased during high-frequency but not low-frequency acupoint stimulation relative to control stimulation. Moreover, decreased theta power was prominent at the FCZ and contralateral right hemisphere frontal (FCC2h) areas during high-frequency simulation.

It was previously reported that subject pain perception combined with the corresponding EEG waveforms could be used to describe the body's systemic neural response to a given stimulation (Kakigi et al. 2005). One study evaluated the statistical relationship between brain activity and the experience of pain induced by GB34 stimulation with intensive light impulses (wavelength, 500–1200 nm) (Lee et al. 2011). EEG data were recorded from sites F(p1) and F(p2). According to the results, the area under the curve of brain waves induced by pain was useful as a proportional indicator of pain perception.

Another study explored the relationship between electrical activity changes measured with EEG and patient experiences during acupuncture using items of the acupuncture sensation questionnaire (Yin et al. 2010). The results indicated that only the group with higher ratings of needle sensation showed significant changes in alpha band EEG powers over the periods before, during, and after needle insertion. Accordingly, acupuncture effects on EEG activity may closely relate to needle sensation in some patients.

Studies of acupuncture on healthy subjects have mainly explored the specificity of acupuncture according to the principles of Traditional Chinese Medicine by examining acupoint specificity, acupuncture sensation, and different responses induced by distinct stimulation methods. However, the findings are difficult to synthesize and even contradictory in many cases due to inter-study differences in experimental design, small sample sizes, and the details of acupoint stimulation.

Studies in patients with indications for acupuncture. Intraoperative transcutaneous acupoint electrical stimulation (TAES) has been reported to improve the sedative effect of propofol, a widely used sedative anesthetic agent (Nayak et al. 2008; Ding et al. 2013). Further, TAES has also been reported to reduce post-operative opioid intake and decrease the incidence side effects related to anesthesia while improving the quality of recovery from anesthesia (Wang et al. 1997, 2014). The mechanism of TAES and its beneficial interactions with anesthetics was investigated in a previous EEG oscillation analysis (Liu et al. 2016). EEG was continuously measured during both light and deep propofol sedation (target-controlled infusion set at 1.0 and 3.0 μg/mL, respectively) in ten patients undergoing surgery. Propofol infusion was maintained for 6 min, and each 6-min period was divided into three 2-min phases. TAES was initiated between 3–4 min after initiation of the propofol infusion. EEG power spectrum changes in different frequency bands (delta, theta, alpha, beta, and gamma) and the coherence of different EEG channels were analyzed. The result showed that after TAES application, EEG power was increased in the alpha and beta bands during light sedation, but was reduced in the delta and beta bands during deep sedation (Fig. 4.4). In addition, the EEG oscillation analysis showed that TEAS increased synchronization at low frequencies and decreased synchronization at high frequencies during light or deep propofol sedation (Fig. 4.5). Accordingly, while this study suggested that TAES might improve the effects of propofol during light sedation, it is hard to conclude that TAES is beneficial in combination with propofol anesthesia without further corroboration of these findings.

Silva and colleagues analyzed the efficacy of TENS for post-mastectomy pain and its ability to produce eletrocortical changes in somatosensory areas (Silva et al. 2014). EEG was recorded in absolute power in the alpha band (8–14 Hz), and pain assessments were conducted before and after TENS intervention. TENS produced decreases in both slow (8–10 Hz) and fast alpha (10–12 Hz) wavebands and led to 88.4% reduction of pain scores. Accordingly, it was concluded that TENS supported the modulation of electrical stimulation in the parietal region and reduced clinical post-mastectomy pain.

In conclusion, EEG is often used to diagnose disorders that influence brain activity, such as epilepsy (Chu et al. 1991; Chu 1992), dementia (Gao et al. 2001), and

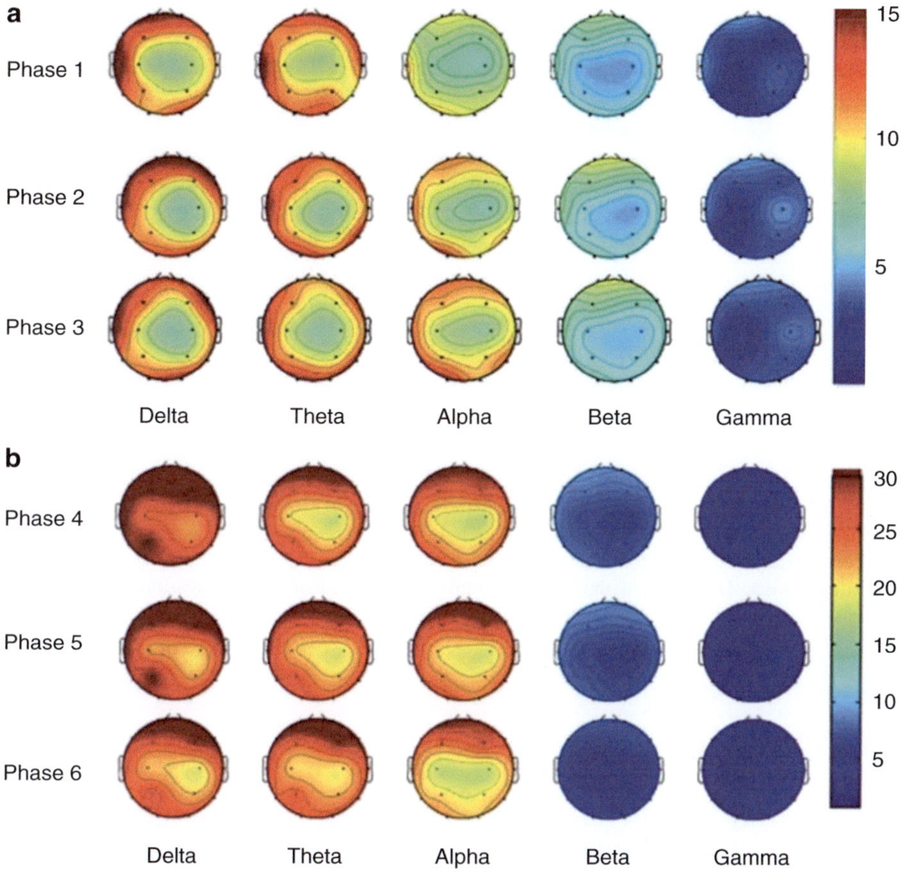

Fig. 4.4 Topoplot of EEG powers in different frequency bands during different phases during (**a**) light propofol sedation and (**b**) deep propofol sedation (Reprint from Liu et al. 2016). Transcutaneous acupoint electrical stimulation was applied during phases 2 and 5

attention-deficit hyperactivity disorder (Arnold 2001). Yet, the number of acupuncture clinical trials using EEG is relatively small. Future studies should employ EEG in the assessment of acupuncture in patients with acupuncture indications in order to better elucidate possible mechanisms of action.

In summary, EEG is a convenient and safe method that is widely used for preclinical and clinical research. Notably, EEG can provide precise temporal dynamic information about the effects and mechanisms of action of acupuncture. A majority of studies to date has focused on evaluating the characteristics of acupuncture in humans and various animal models. However, the conclusions of these studies have been inconsistent; the differences of stimulation acupoints, stimulation types, and experimental design might contribute to the inconformity.

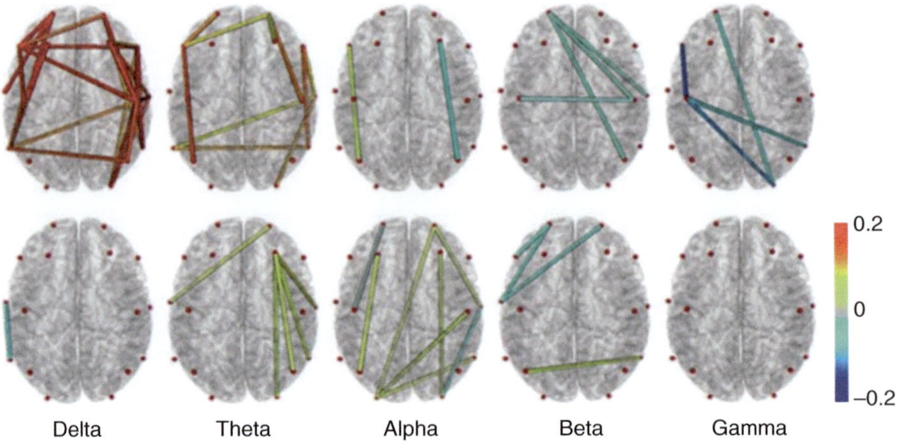

Fig. 4.5 The effects of transcutaneous acupoint electrical stimulation (TAES) on synchronization among EEG channels at different frequency bands during propofol administration at 1 μg/mL (**a**) and 3 μg/mL (**b**) (Reprint from Liu et al. 2016). *Red* nodes indicate cortical electrodes. *Lines* between nodes indicate significant changes in synchronization between the two channels before and after TAES. The color of the line represents the strength of synchronization (*red* indicates increased synchronization and *blue* indicates decreased synchronization)

4.4 Principles of MEG

Neural activity in the brain gives rise to electrical currents that spread in the surrounding volume conductor and produces volume currents that partially reach the surface of the scalp. Volume currents are passive in nature and behave, on a macroscopic scale, according to Ohm's law. Volume currents are generated in response to primary currents, which flow inside of or in the vicinity of neurons (Lutkenhoner 2003). Accordingly, both primary currents and volume currents contribute to magnetic fields measured by MEG. That is, when information is being processed, sufficient current flow can produce a weak magnetic field that can be measured noninvasively using a magnetometer placed on the outside of the skull. However, magnetic fields only reflect activity in the uppermost layer of the brain, the cerebral cortex, which is a 2–4-mm thick sheet of gray matter tissue. Although MEG is a relatively new method of recording, it has already facilitated novel research on the functioning of the human brain and is expected to become increasingly important in the near future as clinical applications for MEG emerge.

Regions of the brain that are activated in response to a given stimulus or during the resting state can be localized based on the observation of magnetic fields using MEG. In this case, a typical MEG signal can be evoked by a tone burst.

4.4.1 Basic Principles of MEG

Sensory stimuli initially activate small pertinent portions of the cortex. This process is associated with primary current generation related to the movement of ions across neuronal membranes according to their chemical concentration gradients. In addition, passive ohmic currents (volume current) are produced in the surrounding medium. This volume current completes the loop of ionic flow so that there is no buildup of charge. Together, primary current and volume current lead to the generation of a magnetic field. If the primary source and surrounding conductivity distribution are known, the resulting magnetic field can be calculated from Maxwell's equations as follows:

$$\nabla \cdot \vec{E} = \frac{\rho}{\varepsilon_0} \tag{4.1}$$

$$\nabla \times \vec{E} = -\frac{\delta \vec{B}}{\delta t} \tag{4.2}$$

$$\nabla \cdot \vec{B} = 0 \tag{4.3}$$

$$\nabla \times \vec{B} = \mu_0 \vec{J} + \mu_0 \varepsilon_0 \frac{\delta \vec{E}}{\delta t} \tag{4.4}$$

where $\vec{E}$ represents the electric field, $\vec{B}$ represents the magnetic field, ρ represents the volume density of free charges, ε_0 represents the mediated rate, and μ_0 represents magnetic permeability.

In certain finite conductor geometries, the volume current causes the generation of an equivalent and opposite field to the primary current. The net external field is then zero. Therefore, MEG can only measure activity from fissures of the cortex. Because all primary sensory areas of the brain (auditory, somatosensory, and visual) are located within fissures, MEG can be used to study functional brain responses to a variety of stimuli.

4.4.1.1 The Current Dipole Source Model

Current dipole is a popular source model in MEG research that is used to approximate the flow of electrical current in small areas. The typical strength of a dipole caused by the synchronous activity of what is likely to be tens of thousands of neurons is 10 nA m. For a single current dipole source, the map of the radial magnetic field B has one maximum and one minimum. The dipole is half of the field extremum at a right angle to the line joining the maximum and minimum. The magnitude, direction, and position of the source can be deduced unambiguously from this map, provided that the dipolar assumption is valid, i.e., the source currents are limited to a small region of the brain. This model provides a basis for the consideration of more complex source constellations. In principle, any conceivable distribution of

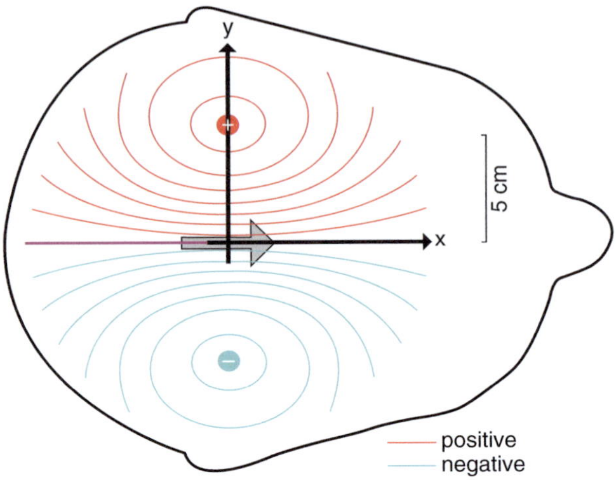

Fig. 4.6 Contours of a human head with a topographical map visualizing the normal component of a magnetic field arising from a current dipole (Lutkenhoner 2003). The dipole (*thick gray arrow*) is located 6 cm below the measurement surface (sphere with a radius of 12 cm). The two field extrema are represented by *filled circles*. The *symbols* indicate the polarity of the magnetic field: + for magnetic flux out of the head and – for magnetic flux into the head (Reprint with permission from Wikswo and Roth 1988)

currents in the brain can be represented in terms of current dipoles. In addition, no more than six parameters are required to define this model: the three coordinates of the dipole location and the three components of the dipole moment. The latter is a vector having the same orientation as the mean current in the source. The length of this vector corresponds to the strength of the current multiplied by a measure of length, which characterizes the mean distance over which the current flows.

The magnetic field arising from a current dipole has a characteristic pattern. To illustrate this point, the contours of the human head are shown in Fig. 4.6. The bulky short arrow represents a current dipole located 6 cm below the measurement surface. This dipole is aligned with the x-axis, which runs from the center of the head to the nasion. The normal component of the magnetic field arising from this dipole is visualized as a topographical map; magnetic flux directed out of the head (positive polarity) is shown in the left hemisphere, whereas magnetic flux directed into the head is shown in the right hemisphere. In between these two hemispheres is the median plane, where the flux is zero. The two field extrema are located in a plane running orthogonal to the median plane through the y-axis.

4.4.2 Measurement of MEG Signal

Compared to potentials recorded at the scalp, which depend on the conductivities of the brain, skull, and scalp, magnetic field is able to pass through intervening tissues unchanged; this means that the head is essentially transparent to magnetic fields.

However, it is known that the magnetic field component perpendicular to the scalp (normal component) is not very sensitive to volume currents. Thus, detailed information about the volume conductor is often dispensable for data analysis. This is one reason why MEG measurements favor the normal component of the magnetic field.

MEG signal is typically measured at a distance of about 2 cm from the scalp using a sensitive superconducting quantum interference device (SQUID) detector (Kim et al. 2014). Because magnetic signals from the brain are extremely weak compared with ambient magnetic-field variations, the elimination of outside disturbances is of utmost importance. For example, the electrical activity of the heart generates a magnetic field that is 2–3 orders of magnitude larger than signals originating from the brain. To this end, the sensitivity of SQUID detectors to external magnetic noise is greatly reduced by proper design of the Aux transformer, a device that facilitates magnetic signal detection by the SQUID. In addition, MEG measurements are usually performed in a magnetically shielded room.

4.4.3 MEG Data Processing

The neural processing of incoming information can be studied by recording responses to sensory stimuli. In many experiments, spontaneous brain activity and incoherent background events can be sources of noise. Thus, signals resulting from many successive stimuli must be averaged to isolate evoked responses. For localization of the active brain area, measurements are made over several sites, typically 20–60 points across the scalp separated by about 3 cm. At each location, the stimulus must be repeated 20–500 times in order to produce an adequate signal-to-noise ratio. This is a potentially tedious and time-consuming procedure that also endangers the reliability of the data: the subject cannot be expected to remain in the same state of vigilance throughout long measurement sessions.

Indeed, the primary drawback of MEG in early studies was the amount of time required to gather sufficient data for topographical field map generation. To minimize the amount of time required, several MEG research groups and companies are already constructing and using multi-SQUID magnetometers. For example, a 24-channel neurogradiometer employing planar gradiometric flux transformers was recently developed to provide accelerated data acquisition.

Another factor seriously influencing the quality of MEG signal is the distance between the source and the center of the head. It is useful to consider the idealized case of a volume conductor with spherical symmetry; for such a volume conductor, the amplitude of the MEG signal does not only decrease with the squared distance between source and measurement site, but is, in addition, proportional to the distance between the source and the center of the sphere (Lutkenhoner 1996). Thus, a source in the center is magnetically silent. In practice, a deep source is not completely silent on MEG, but can be expected to produce a magnetic field that is about one order of magnitude smaller than that of a comparable source located close to the surface of the brain (Menninghaus and Lutkenhoner 1995). There is opportunity for the improvement of this aspect of MEG, but additional studies are required to facilitate this advancement.

4.4.3.1 The Inverse Problem

Given a complete knowledge of currents and a sufficiently realistic volume conductor model, it is relatively easy to calculate the associated magnetic field. This matter is often called the forward problem. However, in practice, the problem is reversed: the magnetic field is given, and the task is to estimate the underlying currents in the brain. Unfortunately, this inverse problem has no unique solution; in principle, each magnetic field has an infinite number of possible interpretations.

When put into use, a single current dipole is rarely a perfect model, which means that at least one additional dipole is required to explain the data. Yet, it is often difficult to ascertain how many additional dipoles are required, given that successively increasing the number of dipoles rarely results in a sharp transition from an insufficient match to an almost perfect match between model and data. In addition, the fact that the number of model parameters often exceeds the number of independent data values is also a problem. To mitigate this situation, several methods have been developed, such as the parametric method, which assumes that a source consists of a few current dipoles, and the imaging method, which is based on the idea of a continuous distribution of main currents throughout the whole brain (Baillet et al. 2001). Each method has its specific advantages and disadvantages (Kaufman et al. 1990).

4.4.3.2 MEG Resolution Issues

The time resolution of MEG is better than 1 ms, and the spatial or imaging resolution is (under favorable circumstances) 2–3 mm for sources in the human brain. Spatial resolution is defined as the spatial limit (distance) between two sources that permits the independent resolution of each source. However, in practice, it is not impossible to characterize the spatial resolution of a given method using a single number, since numerous factors need be taken into consideration (Supek and Aine 1993). It has been suggested that, as a rule of thumb, two sources can only be resolved and separated if the intersource distance is at least of the same order of magnitude as the distance between the sources and measurement locations (Tan et al. 1990). This rule is consistent with the finding that it is difficult to calculate the spatial extent of a source from MEG measurements whenever the source-to-coil distance is much larger than the dimensions of the source (Wikswo and Roth 1988).

Spatial or imaging resolution is not to be confused with localizing resolution, which refers to the accuracy with which a particular source can be localized by a given method (Dale and Halgren 2001; Florin and Baillet 2015). Although the localizing resolution has no principle limitation, limitations in practice are imposed by noise in the data as well as model inaccuracies. The localizing resolution of MEG under favorable circumstances makes it useful for identifying functional landmarks in the brain, which can be of value in stereotactic and functional neurosurgery (Orrison 1999).

Imaging methods (discussed in the previous section) tend to identify sources as relatively widespread, even when the sources themselves are small or relatively specific. This behavior can be characterized by the point spread function, which describes how activity at a distinct point in the brain affects estimated activity in other locations (Liu et al. 2002). Another measure characterizing the spatial resolution of a method is the resolution field (Lutkenhoner 2001; Liu et al. 2002); the resolution field specifies how activity estimated for a certain point in the brain is affected by activities at other locations. The resolution field is not only defined for imaging methods but also for parametric methods.

4.4.4 Characterization of MEG Data in Different Frequency Bands

MEG data is collected in several different frequency bands; that is, analyses are usually performed for the most commonly used frequency bands in order to facilitate comparisons with other studies. These bands include the delta (0.5–4 Hz), theta (4–8 Hz), alpha (8–12 Hz), beta (13–30 Hz), and gamma (30–45 Hz) frequency bands (Siebenhuhner et al. 2013; Bajo et al. 2015; Kotini and Anninos 2016). Data in each frequency band provides information about different characteristics of human brain functions.

The delta frequency band has a typical voltage amplitude between 20 and 200 μV and represents the deep sleep state of the human brain. By contrast, the theta frequency band has a typical voltage amplitude between 100–150 μV and represents the general sleep state. For the alpha frequency band, the typical voltage amplitude is between 20–100 μV, and this band represents the quiet and waking states of the human brain. Finally, the beta frequency band has a typical voltage amplitude between 5–20 μV and represents the activated state. Among these frequency bands, the beta frequency band is most closely related to REM sleep, while delta and theta frequency bands are usually involved in non-REM sleep.

Studies of spontaneous brain activity are greatly benefited by multisensor array recording. In evoked response experiments, data from several sites measured at different times can be combined fairly safely, whereas this is not possible for recordings of spontaneous activity (where every event is unique). On the other hand, many spontaneous brain signals with sufficient strength can be recorded without averaging.

The appearance of MEG data from an awake subject resembles that of EEG data: the parieto-occipital areas show 8–12-Hz alpha activities that are dampened by opening of the eyes. In the first study of human magnetic rhythms, a phase reversal was observed between signals measured from the right and left hemispheres, and the oscillating source currents were suggested to be parallel to the longitudinal fissure between the hemispheres. Chapman et al. used the relative covariance method with an electric reference at the vertex and the resultant map showed two extrema, with one at each parieto-occipital area. The distribution agreed with a two-dipole model, with the sources in the vicinity of the calcarine fissure (the site of the primary visual cortex), symmetric with respect to the cortical midline, and 4–6 cm beneath the scalp. The magnetic a signal was selectively suppressed on one side by independent stimulation of the left or right visual field. Kaufman et al. similarly demonstrated that occipital magnetic activity was suppressed for about 1 s during a visual memory task (Kaufman et al. 1990); this effect was found by monitoring the average field variance at the frequency. These MEG results confirmed sources of the alpha rhythm in humans that were only previously detected by microelectrode studies in animals.

4.4.5 Methods for MEG Data Analysis

To be considered as functional imaging techniques, EEG and MEG require careful pre- and post-processing of scalp recording data in order to provide a reliable functional map of brain activity (He et al. 2011). Advanced models and numerical methods rely on trustworthy physiological assumptions, exploring data in their full spatial, temporal, and spectral ranges (Lin et al. 2004). Indeed, the brain is a complex system that exhibits different properties at various spatial and temporal scales (Lina et al. 2014). Accordingly, a variety of methods have been developed and adopted for the processing and analysis of MEG data.

4.4.5.1 Partial Least Squares (PLS)

MEG is a neuroimaging modality that captures neural activity with a high degree of temporal specificity. The PLS analysis is a multivariate framework that can be used to isolate distributed spatiotemporal patterns of neural activity that differentiate groups or cognitive tasks in order to relate neural activity to behavior and capture large-scale network interactions. Therefore, the MEG imaging modality and the PLS framework are complementary and together offer great potential for network discovery and analysis. A number of recent studies have demonstrated the benefits of a combined MEG-PLS approach for the study of a wide range of cognitive tasks, including learning and facial recognition and processing, as well as a number of physiological and pathological states including healthy development, healthy aging, traumatic brain injury, and autism spectrum disorders.

A recent paper introduced [MEG]PLS as a platform that streamlines MEG data preprocessing (Cheung et al. 2016), source reconstruction, and PLS analysis in a single unified framework. [MEG]PLS facilitates MRI preprocessing, including segmentation and co-registration; MEG preprocessing, including filtering, epoching, and artifact correction; MEG sensor analysis in both time and frequency domains; and MEG source analysis, including multiple head models and beam-forming algorithms and combines these with a suite of PLS analyses. In this framework, PLS facilitates multivariate exploration and network discovery using MEG data. The application of PLS to source-reconstructed MEG data takes advantage of the rich spatial and temporal information contained in MEG signal, allowing investigators to derive distributed spatiotemporal patterns of neural activity and relate these patterns to experimental manipulations and/or behavior.

A principal strength of PLS is its data-driven nature, which makes it ideal for exploratory analyses in which the investigator has no strong hypothesis about the differentiation of groups or conditions, or about the specific spatiotemporal expression of a particular effect. In summary, [MEG]PLS is a tool designed to help investigators explore MEG data from a multivariate perspective and to better address experimental questions about distributed activity patterns and network function. That is, [MEG]PLS allows investigators to easily transition from preprocessing to source reconstruction to PLS analysis and offers investigators the flexibility to adapt analysis streams to their data and experimental questions.

4.4.5.2 Principal Component Analysis (PCA)

PCA is a statistical procedure that uses an orthogonal transformation to convert a set of observations of possibly correlated variables into a set of values of linearly uncorrelated variables known as principal components. This transformation is defined in such a way that the first principal component has the largest possible variance. Principal components are orthogonal because they are the eigenvectors of the covariance matrix, which is symmetric. Of note, PCA is sensitive to the relative scaling of the original variables.

PCA is mostly adopted as a tool for exploratory data analysis and to construct predictive models (Siebenhuhner et al. 2013). PCA can be performed by eigenvalue decomposition of a data covariance matrix or singular value decomposition of a data matrix, usually after mean centering (and normalizing or using Z-scores) the data matrix for each attribute (Abdi and Williams 2010). The results of a PCA are usually discussed in terms of component scores, sometimes called factor scores (the transformed variable values corresponding to a particular data point), and loadings (the weight by which each standardized original variable should be multiplied to obtain the component score).

PCA can be considered as fitting an n-dimensional ellipsoid to a given data set, where each axis of the ellipsoid represents a principal component. If an axis of the ellipse is small, then the variance along that axis is also small; accordingly, by omitting that axis and its corresponding principal component from the data set representation, only a commensurately small amount of information is lost. To determine the axes of the ellipse, the mean of each variable must first be subtracted from the data set in order to center the data around the origin. Then, the covariance matrix of the data is computed and the eigenvalues and corresponding eigenvectors of this covariance matrix are calculated. Next, the resultant set of eigenvectors is orthogonalized and normalized to yield unit vectors. Once this is done, each of the mutually orthogonal, unit eigenvectors can be interpreted as an axis of the ellipsoid fitted to the data. The proportion of the variance that each eigenvector represents can be calculated by dividing the eigenvalue corresponding to that eigenvector by the sum of all eigenvalues.

PCA is the simplest of true eigenvector-based multivariate analyses. Often, its operation can be thought of as revealing the internal structure of the data in a way that best explains the variance in the data. If a multivariate data set is visualized as a set of coordinates in a high-dimensional data space (1 axis per variable), PCA can supply the user with a lower-dimensional picture, projection, or "shadow" of the object when viewed from its most informative viewpoint. However, this is done by using only the first few principal components, such that the dimensionality of the transformed data is reduced.

Notably, PCA is closely related to factor analysis. However, factor analysis typically incorporates more domain-specific assumptions about the underlying structure and solves the eigenvectors of a slightly different matrix.

4.4.5.3 Root Mean Square (RMS)

In statistics, the RMS (also known as the quadratic mean) is defined as the square root of the arithmetic mean of the squares of a set of numbers. The root mean square is a particular case of the generalized mean with the exponent 2. In the case of a set of n values $\{x_1, x_2, x_{3t}, x_n\}$, the RMS is as follows:

$$RMS = \sqrt{\frac{x_1^2 + x_2^2 + \cdots + x_n^2}{n}} \tag{4.5}$$

In one previous MEG study, RMS values were calculated for each subject over all sensor channels for the averaged data sets of the standard, deviant, and difference (deviant minus standard) data sets (Lappe et al. 2016).

Compared to the mean value, the error of actual experimental results contains both negative and positive values. Because RMS eliminates the sign effect when the squared error is calculated, it better reflects the discreteness of the error of the experimental results.

4.4.5.4 Independent Component Analysis (ICA)

In MEG signal processing, ICA is a computational method for separating a given multivariate signal into additive subcomponents. That is, ICA is used to decompose independent patterns of brain or artifact activity that are linearly mixed into the functional data. This is accomplished by assuming that the subcomponents are non-Gaussian signals that are statistically independent from each other. ICA is accordingly a special case of blind source separation. An important question is thus whether it is possible to separate contributing sources from the observed total signal. When the statistical independence assumption is correct, blind ICA separation of a mixed signal yields very good results. ICA is also used to analyze signals that are not supposed to be generated by mixing for analytical purposes.

ICA of short-time Fourier transforms of resting-state MEG or EEG signals has been proposed as a method to identify sources of intrinsic rhythmic activity within the cortex. A recent study adopted ICA to analyze MEG signals in this manner (Mantini et al. 2011). In the work by Mantini et al., MEG recordings were decomposed by ICA into artifact and brain components. Several ICA algorithms were assessed for utility in the analysis of MEG resting-state data.

Accordingly, ICA has been shown to be a valuable tool for the attenuation of artifacts and noise in MEG and EEG analyses (Mantini et al. 2008) (Fig. 4.7) and for the investigation of brain source activity (Barati et al. 2006).

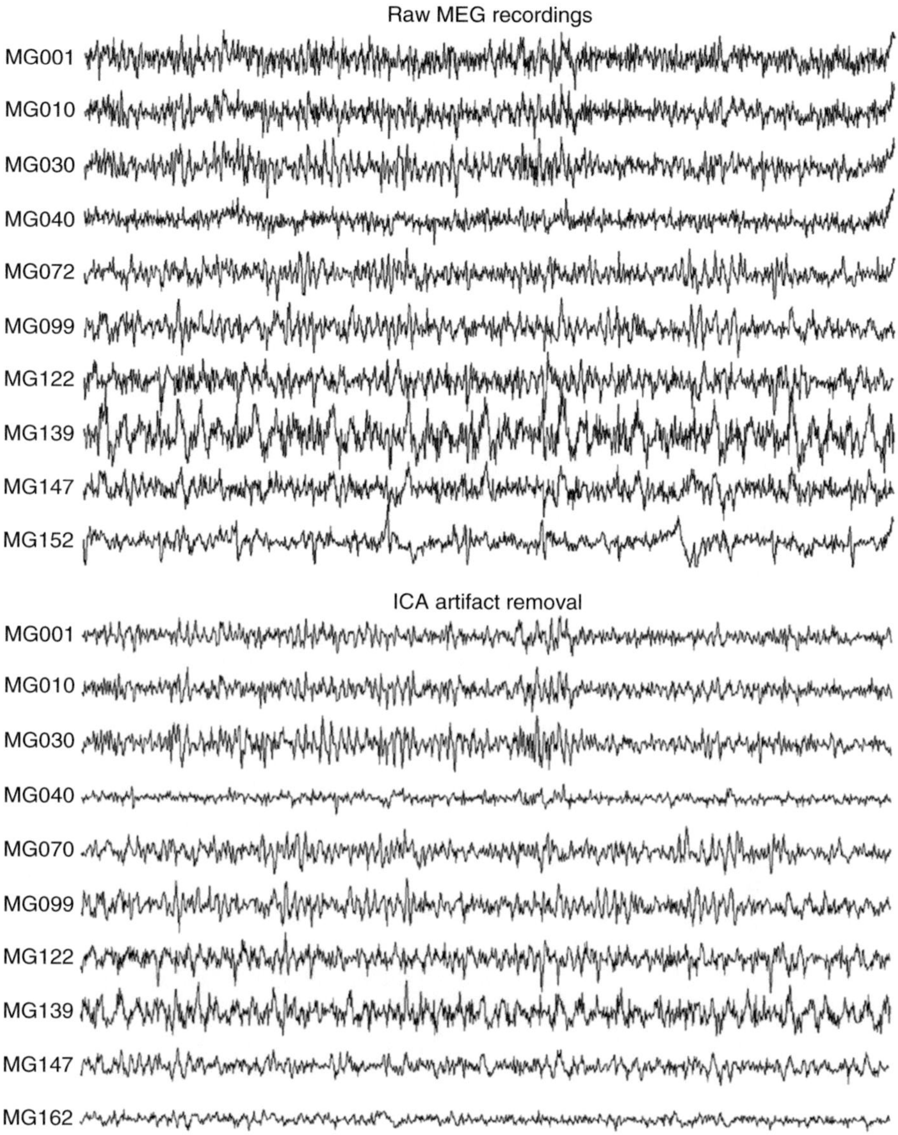

Fig. 4.7 Artifact-free MEG traces corresponding to the raw signals presented in *top panel*. Signals reconstructed by means of ICA (*bottom panel*) (Reprint with permission from Mantini et al. 2008)

4.4.5.5 Signal Space Separation (SSS)

SSS is a new method for removing external disturbances and movement artifacts, calculating virtual signals, and performing movement correction and direct current measurements for MEG data. SSS efficiently exploits the fact that the number of channels in modern multichannel MEG devices exceeds the number of degrees of freedom of the measurable magnetic fields (Taulu et al. 2004). Using SSS, any measured signal can be uniquely decomposed into separate components representing the biomagnetic signals arising from inside of the array and the external interference signals arising from outside of the array. Two studies have adopted this method for the processing of MEG data (Miozzo et al. 2014; Florin and Baillet 2015). SSS greatly improves the quality of MEG data without requiring extensive user intervention, which is a particularly important feature in the clinical context. Moreover, SSS allows measurements with varying interference sources in the environment and even in moving subjects with moderate magnetic impurities or implants.

4.4.5.6 Multiple Linear Regressions

In statistics, linear regression is an approach for modeling the relationship between a scalar dependent variable y and one or more explanatory variables (or independent variables) denoted by x. The case of one explanatory variable is called simple linear regression, whereas cases with more than one explanatory variable are called multiple linear regression. Like all regression analyses, linear regression focuses on the conditional probability distribution of y given x, rather than on the joint probability distribution of y and x.

Linear regression models are often fitted using the least squares approach, but they may also be fitted in other ways, such as by minimizing the lack of fit in some other norm or by minimizing a penalized version of the least squares loss function as in ridge regression and lasso. Conversely, the least squares approach can be used to fit models that are not linear models. Of note, although the terms "least squares" and "linear model" are closely linked, they are not synonymous.

The simplest case of a single scalar predictor variable x and a single scalar response variable y is known as simple linear regression. The inclusion of multiple and/or vector-valued predictor variables (denoted by X) is known as a multiple or multivariable linear regression. Nearly all real-world regression models involve multiple predictors, and basic descriptions of linear regression are often phrased in terms of the multiple regression model. It is important to note, however, that in these cases the response variable y is still a scalar.

Multiple linear regression has been used in some MEG studies (Tan et al. 1990). For example, a multiple linear regression approach was used to investigate the early effects of variables specifically related to visual, semantic, and phonological processing on picture naming in one MEG analysis. This study combined a multiple linear aggression with distributed minimum-norm source estimation and a region-of-interest analysis. The results demonstrated that multiple linear regression was sensitive to the early effects of multiple psycholinguistic variables.

4.4.5.7 Analysis of Variance (ANOVA)

ANOVA describes a collection of statistical models and associated procedures used to analyze differences among group means. In the context of an ANOVA, the observed variance for a particular variable is partitioned into components attributable to different sources of variation. In its simplest form, ANOVA provides a statistical test of whether or not the means of several groups are equal and therefore adapts the *t*-test to evaluate more than two groups. On this premise, the ANOVA is conceptually similar to multiple two-sample *t*-tests but is less conservative and therefore suited to address a wide range of practical problems.

ANOVA can be used to study the effects of multiple factors. When an experiment includes observations at all combinations of levels of each factor, it is termed factorial. Factorial experiments are more efficient than a series of single-factor experiments, and efficiency increases as the number of factors increases. Consequently, factorial designs are heavily used in research.

Use of the ANOVA to study the effects of multiple factors has some complications. In a three-way ANOVA with factors x, y, and z, the ANOVA model includes terms for the main effects (x, y, z) and terms for interactions (xy, xz, yz, xyz). All terms require hypothesis testing. Larger numbers of interaction terms increase the risk of a false-positive result. Fortunately, high-order interactions are known to be rare. The ability to detect interactions is a major advantage of multiple-factor ANOVAs.

In one recent study, an ANOVA analysis was applied to test relationships between clinical characteristics (e.g., age, disease duration, pain type, and frequency) and MEG parameters (source location and magnetic source power) as measured by Spearman correlation coefficients (Kim et al. 2014).

Finally, the ANOVA is also used for the analysis of comparative experiments, in which only the difference in outcomes is of interest. The statistical significance of the experiment is determined by a ratio of two variances. This ratio is independent of several possible alterations (e.g., adding a constant or multiplying all observations by a constant) to the experimental observations. Accordingly, ANOVA results are independent of constant bias and scaling errors as well as the units used for observation expression.

4.5 Comparison Between the MEG and EEG Techniques

The use of modern noninvasive imaging techniques to investigate the structure and function of the brain is an increasingly popular and important area of neuroscience research. Some techniques such as EEG have the advantage of a high spatial resolution, whereas others such as MEG have low spatial resolution but high temporal resolution.

EEG, the measurement of electric potential differences on the scalp, is a widely applied method with long-standing clinical use. MEG is in fact closely related to EEG. In both methods, the measured signals are generated by the same synchronized neuronal activity in the brain. Of note, these electrical events typically last from one to several tens of milliseconds. Moreover, both EEG and MEG provide a projection of the primary current distribution on respective lead fields, so they are formally on equal footing. In addition, they both measure weighted integrals of the primary current distribution. The temporal resolution of MEG and EEG is in the millisecond range, which is orders of magnitude better than other methods. Thus, MEG and EEG can both be used to monitor rapid changes in cortical activity that reflect ongoing signal processing in the brain. A very important advantage of MEG and EEG is that they are completely noninvasive.

Although both MEG and EEG have low spatial resolutions, MEG has better spatial accuracy than EEG, within a few millimeters under favorable conditions. This is because electrical potentials measured on the scalp are often influenced by various heterogeneities that complicate accurate determination of the activated area. By contrast, a magnetic field is mainly produced by currents that flow in a macroscopically homogeneous intracranial space. Moreover, because of the poor electrical conductivity of bone, irregular currents in the skull and on the scalp are weak and can be ignored as contributors to the external magnetic field.

While the capabilities of EEG and MEG continue to be evaluated in clinical and research settings, several important differences can be summarized as follows:

1. MEG is only sensitive to the tangential current component, while EEG detects all primary current components.
2. The interpretation of EEG signals requires precise knowledge of the thicknesses and conductivities of the tissues in the head.
3. The instrumentation necessary for MEG is more sophisticated and more expensive than that for EEG.
4. MEG measurements can be accomplished more quickly than EEG measurements, since electrode contact with the scalp need not be established.
5. Subjects have to remain still during MEG measurements, whereas EEG permits telemetric and long-term recordings.

Cohen et al. also provided comparison between MEG and EEG in their discussion (Cohen et al. 1990). The authors purported that MEG is slightly more accurate than EEG for localizing a tangential dipole source, that is, cerebral electrical activity. In the study, the authors almost had no opportunities to form artificial current dipoles to observe abnormal cerebral activity; rather, the precise position of each source was determined using roentgenograms. A comparison between the capacities of MEG and EEG was thus possible. Electrical fields were measured with 16 scalp electrodes, and magnetic fields were measured with a single-channel SQUID magnetometer at 16 cranial sites. Locations of the test dipoles were calculated on the basis of MEG and EEG measurements and reported with 8-mm and 10-mm average error for source location, respectively. The paper was criticized by Hari et al. (1991) and Williamson (1991) on methodological grounds as follows:

1. The magnetic field was inappropriately sampled.
2. The dipoles were 16 mm in length, although they were assumed to be point-like in the data analysis. This does not only affect the EEG results but also has the potential to obscure possible differences between the capabilities of MEG and EEG.

3. Nearly radial current dipoles were used as test sources. While these dipoles are optimal for EEG, they are barely detectable by MEG. As a result, the signal-to-noise ratio for MEG was considerably lower than that for EEG.
4. Twice as many signals were averaged for EEG than for MEG, which gave an advantage to EEG in the comparison.
5. No attempt to fit a spherical model to the local curvature of the head was reported. This alone may have caused uncertainty comparable to the total reported error.
6. No error estimates were given for the true source locations as determined from roentgenograms.

In summary, it can be considered that EEG and MEG are complementary techniques for localizing and assessing functional brain activity. The best results are ultimately obtained by combining information from both techniques.

4.6 MEG Studies of Acupuncture in Humans

Acupuncture is an ancient East Asian healing modality that has been in use for more than 2000 years. Unfortunately, its mechanisms of action are not well understood, and accordingly there exists controversy regarding its clinical efficacy. Acupuncture needling often evokes complex somatosensory sensations that may modulate the cognitive/affective perception of pain, suggesting that acupuncture effects might be detectable in supporting neural networks. Modern neuroimaging techniques such as MEG provide a means to safely map the neurophysiological correlates of acupuncture in humans (Dhond et al. 2007a, b), providing a “when” for acupuncture effects during task performance on a millisecond time scale. Accordingly, MEG has the potential to produce valuable insights into the functional mechanisms by which acupuncture exerts clinical effects.

Of note, MEG recordings primarily reflect postsynaptic potentials in the dendrites of pyramidal cells within the neocortex. As aforementioned, MEG is more sensitive to superficial sources of synaptic activity than deep sources of activity given that the strength of a neuronal magnetic field decreases as a function of distance from the source. Therefore, MEG can primarily inform the ability of acupuncture to exert its therapeutic effects by modulating a distributed network of superficial brain areas involved in sensory, autonomic, and cognitive/affective processing. Neuroimaging evidence for the effects of acupuncture in the brain is discussed in detail in the sections below.

4.6.1 Effects of Acupuncture at Network Hubs in the Human Brain

Acupuncture has been proposed to have significant modulatory effects on the brain’s default mode network (DMN). One recent study used fMRI and MEG to illustrate how internal brain resting networks are modulated by acupuncture and speculated about the underlying physiological processes (You et al. 2013). A partial correlation analysis was

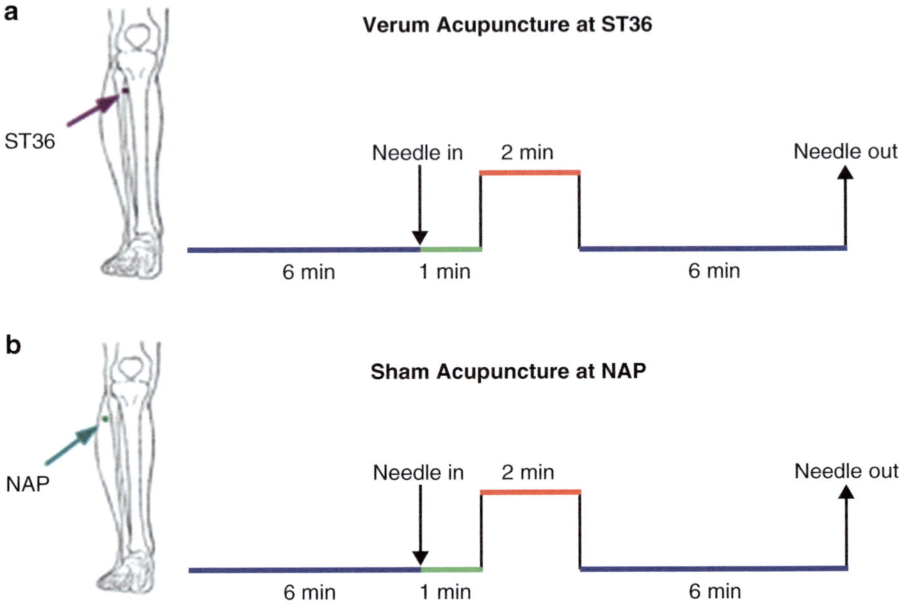

Fig. 4.8 Experimental paradigm (Reprint from You et al. 2013). (**a**) Acupuncture stimulation was performed at ST36 on the right leg (Zusanli, arrow pointing to the *dark pink dot*) or (**b**) at a nearby non-acupoint on the right leg (NAP, arrow pointing to *dark cyan dot*). The *red* lines refer to needling, the *green* lines represent needle insertion without acupuncture manipulation, and the *blue* lines indicate 6-min resting states or post-acupuncture resting states

adopted to estimate intrinsic functional connectivity and network hub configurations in order to explore whether or not band-specific DMN hub configurations were spatiotemporally affected by true acupuncture at ST39 versus acupuncture at a nearby non-meridian acupoint (NAP). The experimental paradigm is shown in Fig. 4.8.

Moreover, based on previous investigations showing band-specific effects of acupuncture on functional connectivity in the whole-brain network, modulation was explored in the delta (0.5–4 Hz), theta (4–8 Hz), alpha (8–13 Hz), beta (13–30 Hz), and gamma frequency bands (30–48 Hz). For psychophysical responses, the prevalence of subjective deqi sensations was expressed as a percentage (Fig. 4.9). In general, all sensations except for coolness were more prevalent in response to ST36 acupuncture than NAP acupuncture.

With regard to band-specific DMN hub configurations, a pairwise functional connectivity analysis between eight core brain regions within the DMN were evaluated for each of the five conventional frequency bands before and after acupuncture. A summary of the results is shown in Table 4.1.

This study demonstrated that acupuncture produced differential effects on DMN hub configurations in each of the five conventional frequency bands following acupuncture at ST36 versus NAP. The results highlighted the role of the PCC as a DMN hub within the theta, alpha, and beta bands and provided evidence for acupoint specificity at this hub using MEG.

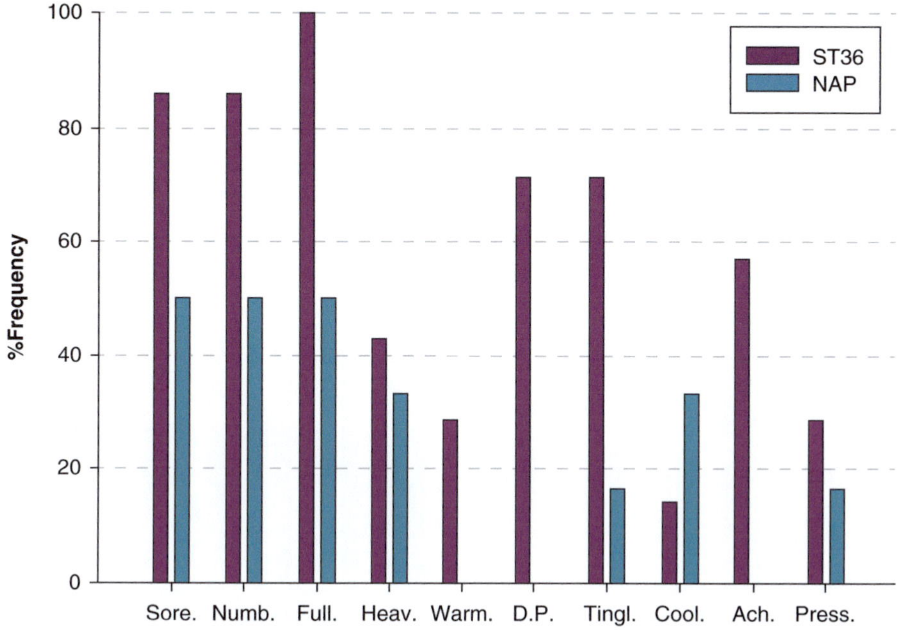

Fig. 4.9 The percentage of subjects that reported different sensations in response to acupuncture at ST36 and a nearby non-acupoint (NAP) (Reprint from You et al. 2013). *Ach* aching, *Cool* coolness, *DP* dull pain, *Full* fullness, *Heav* heaviness, *Numb* numbness, *Press* pressure, *Sore* soreness, *Tingl* tingling, *Warm* warmth (Reprint from You et al. 2013)

Table 4.1 Default mode network hub configurations in five frequency bands, respectively, during the resting state (REST), following sham acupuncture (NAP) or verum acupuncture (ST36) (Reprint from You et al. 2013)

	Conditions		
Frequency band	REST	NAP	ST36
Delta	PCC, IPL	PCC, MTG	PCC, SFG
Theta	PCC	PCC, STG	MFG, STG, SFG
Alpha	PCC, ACC, STG, SFG	PCC, ACC, STG, SFG, MFG	STG, SFG
Beta	PCC, ACC, SFG	PCC, ACC, SFG	ACC, SFG
Gamma	PCC	PCC, ACC	PCC, STG

ACC anterior cingulate cortex, *AG* angular gyrus, *Hem* hemisphere, *IPL* inferior parietal lobule, *L* left, *MFG* medial frontal gyrus, *MTG* middle temporal gyrus, *PCC* posterior cingulate cortex/precuneus, *R* right, *SFG* superior frontal gyrus, *STG* superior temporal gyrus

4.6.2 Effects of Acupuncture on Network Functional Connectivity in the Human Brain

Both traditional literature and clinical data have indicated that the modulatory effects of acupuncture largely depend on the specificity of different acupoints. Another previous study by You and colleagues used MEG to explore whether ST36

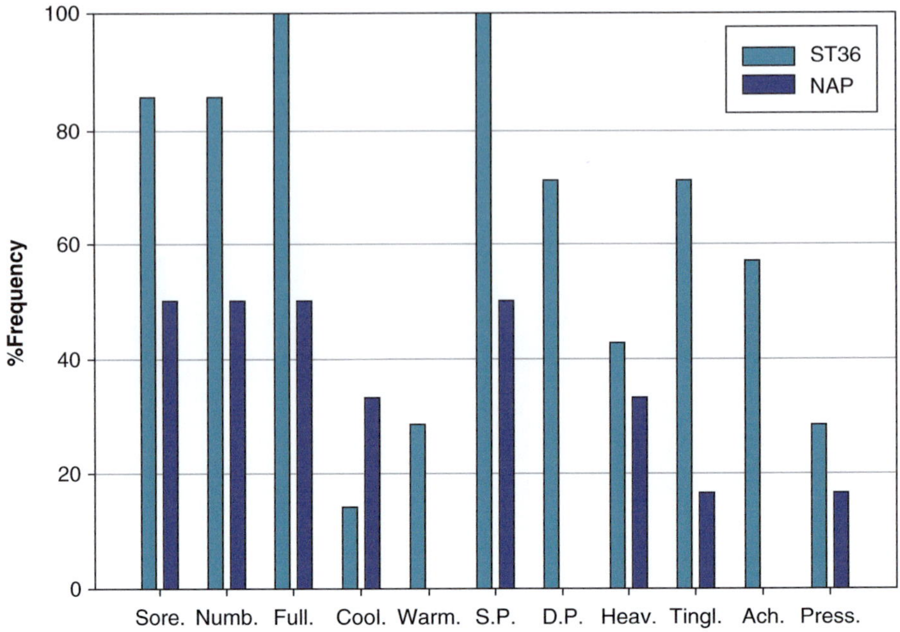

Fig. 4.10 The percentage of subjects that reported different sensations in response to acupuncture at ST36 and a nearby non-acupoint (NAP) (Reprint from You et al. 2012). *Ach* aching, *Cool* coolness, *DP* dull pain, *Full* fullness, *Heav* heaviness, *Numb* numbness, *Press* pressure, *Sore* soreness, *Tingl* tingling, *Warm* warmth (You et al. 2012)

acupuncture versus NAP acupuncture would evoke divergent functional connectivity alterations within the five conventional frequency bands. Averaging was conducted to obtain local and remote connectivity. Once again, deqi sensations were assessed, and all sensations except for coolness were more prevalent in response to ST36 acupuncture than NAP acupuncture (Fig. 4.10).

For the analysis of functional connectivity, temporal correlations of signals for each condition before and after acupuncture were computed for every pair of MEG channels in each frequency band and then grouped into local and long-distance couplings. The grand averaged local and long-distance couplings for each condition in each group were calculated for further statistical analysis. In both acupuncture groups, enhancements in functional connectivity were predominantly observed within the delta band (0.5–4 Hz). In the beta band (13–30 Hz), both groups displayed increased left parieto-occipital connectivity, whereas in the gamma band (30–48 Hz), shared patterns of long- and short-distance interactivity alterations were observed. No significant alterations in functional connectivity were observed in the theta (4–8 Hz) and alpha (8–13 Hz) bands (Fig. 4.11).

Although You et al. observed significant functional connectivity alterations primarily in the delta, beta, and gamma bands, some distinct patterns were observed in response to ST36 versus NAP acupuncture. One intriguing finding was increased

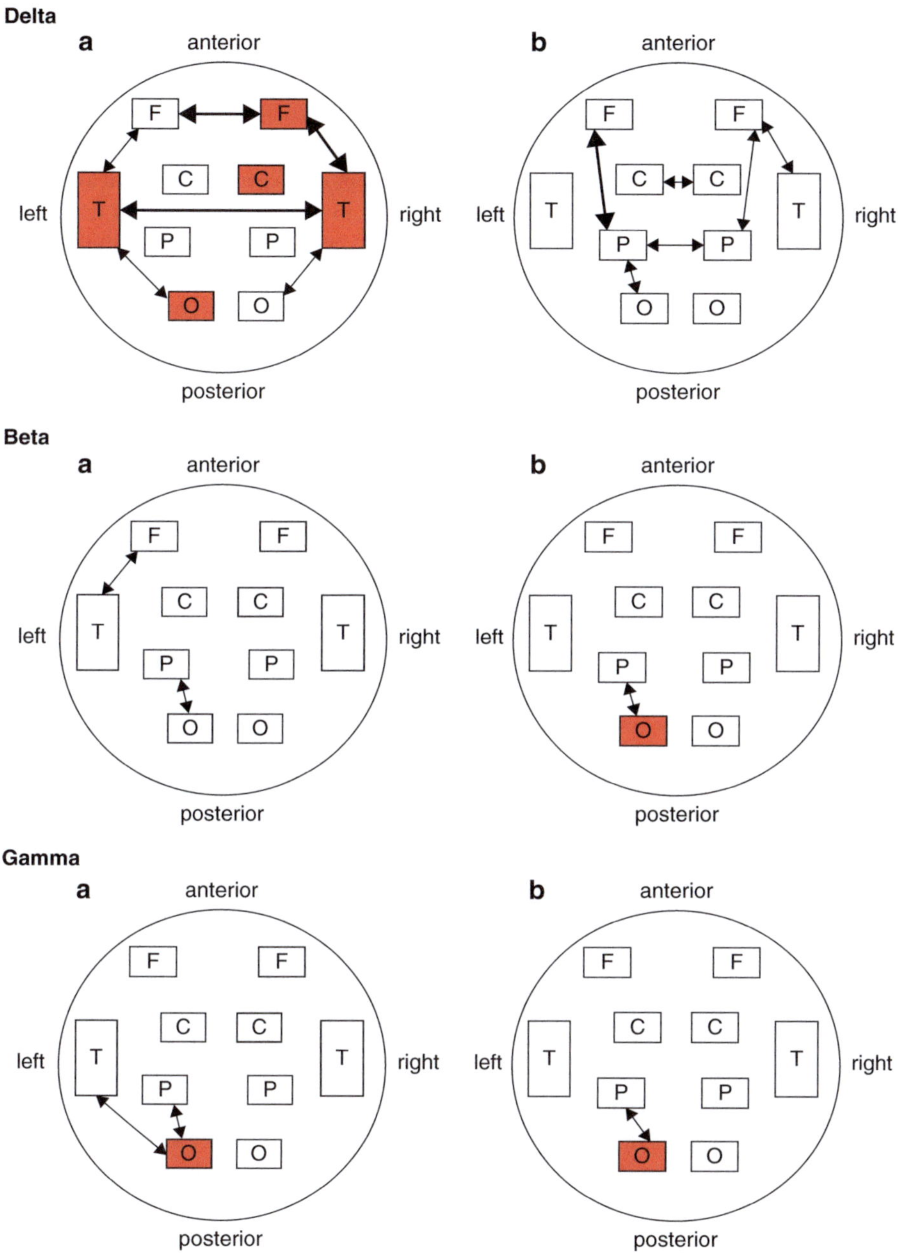

Fig. 4.11 Schematic illustration of BLP correlation alterations for the delta, beta, and gamma bands in the (**a**) ST36 stimulation group and (**b**) nearby non-acupoint (NAP) stimulation group (Reprint from You et al. 2012). Lines correspond to significant correlation changes induced by acupuncture and squares indicate significant changes in local signal correlation (*red*, local increase in signal correlation following acupuncture; *thin line*, $P < 0.05$; *thick line*, $P < 0.01$; paired *t*-test)

connectivity in the left temporal cortex within the delta, theta, and gamma bands after ST36 acupuncture. By contrast, both acupuncture groups presented somewhat shared alteration patterns in the beta and gamma frequency bands in the parietal and occipital regions. These findings suggest that sham acupuncture is also capable of modulating the resting-state network. Moreover, increases in functional connectivity may provide a neurological basis to partly support the clinical observation that acupuncture at non-meridian points can also provide partial analgesia in chronic pain. In conclusion, there are significant opportunities for the implementation EEG and MEG research for the elucidation of acupuncture mechanisms. Studies such as those by You and colleagues can provide a new perspective on the clinical utility of acupuncture and further inform the specificity of acupoint effects on neural activity.

4.7 Summary

The high-resolution spatiotemporal imaging of brain activity requires the integration of information from multiple imaging modalities (Dale and Halgren 2001). However, the spatial resolution of MEG is far coarser than that of functional MRI (Stokes et al. 2015). MRI provides accurate anatomical imaging of the brain with millimeter resolution and is accordingly an outstanding resource for spatial information. Moreover, the time course of MRI signal is roughly a low-pass filtered expression of the total neural activity (Logothetis et al. 2001). Thus, the signals measured by MEG and fMRI have a common physiological basis. To this end, the combination of fMRI techniques with MEG and/or EEG has significant potential benefits. Provided that the coordinate systems for MEG and MRI have been aligned, one can superimpose the locations of brain activity as determined by MEG on that obtained using MRI (George et al. 1989). High-quality anatomical images allow the use of individually shaped realistic conductor models. However, there are some serious practical difficulties that complicate the combination of MEG or EEG and MRI. For example, reliable automatic segmentation of the shape of the brain from MRI is a vital problem, as present techniques require a human operator. With an outline of the structure of interest at hand, it is relatively easy to construct the corresponding triangulation needed for boundary element modeling.

In addition, many methodological problems of multimodal integration are still unsolved (Lutkenhoner 2003). One situation that seems to be underestimated is that the brain structures identified by fMRI are generally activated in an unknown temporal order. Therefore, it is difficult to determine which brain activities observed on fMRI contribute to MEG signal in a given latency range. Improper assumptions about the contributing brain areas have the inevitable consequence that MEG signals are analyzed using a model with inadequate structure (an insufficient number of sources). Severe misinterpretations could result not only from the under-modeling of spatiotemporal MEG data but also from the over-modeling of data (the use of an overly complex source model) (Supek and Aine 1997).

Based on the above issues, a straightforward multimodal synthesis of fMRI source spatial structure and MEG temporal information is predisposed to failure in many situations. Nevertheless, the analysis of MEG data in the context of fMRI data would undoubtedly improve the likelihood of determining accurate sources and at least provide a finite list of candidate sources. In principle, possible combinations of sources explaining a given data set could also be tested; however, new approaches are required to address problematic situations such as cases in which different combinations of sources can explain data with equal plausibility, i.e., the differences between models are small compared to the noise. Moreover, even if the exact source locations are known, an unreasonably high signal-to-noise ratio may be required to separate their respective activities.

In summary, the inverse problem can be partially resolved by incorporating complementary information to restrict the set of possible source configurations. With the assumption that MEG mainly reflects activity in the tangential component of cortical currents, one could, at least in principle, extract the geometry of the cortex from MR images and use the result as a constraint in source estimation procedures.

References

Abdi H, Williams LJ. Principal component analysis. Wiley Interdiscip Rev Comput Stat. 2010;2(4):433–59.

Arai YC, Ushida T, Matsubara T, et al. The influence of acupressure at extra 1 acupuncture point on the spectral entropy of the EEG and the LF/HF ratio of heart rate variability. Evid Based Complement Alternat Med. 2011;2011:503698.

Arnold LE. Alternative treatments for adults with attention-deficit hyperactivity disorder (ADHD). Ann N Y Acad Sci. 2001;931:310–41.

Baillet S, Mosher JC, Leahy RM. Electromagnetic brain mapping. IEEE Signal Process Mag. 2001;18:14–30.

Bajo R, Pusil S, Lopez ME, et al. Scopolamine effects on functional brain connectivity: a pharmacological model of Alzheimer's disease. Sci Rep. 2015;5:9748.

Barati G, Sigismondi R, Zappasodi F, et al. Functional source separation from magnetoencephalographic signals. Hum Brain Mapp. 2006;27:925–34.

Bickford RD. Electroencephalography. In: Adelman G, editor. Encyclopedia of neuroscience. Cambridge: Birkhauser; 1987. p. 371–3.

Caton R. The electric currents of the brain. Br Med J. 1875;2:278.

Chang S, Chang ZG, Li SJ, et al. Effects of acupuncture at Neiguan (PC 6) on electroencephalogram. Chin J Physiol. 2009;52(1):1–7.

Chen AC, Liu FJ, Wang L, et al. Mode and site of acupuncture modulation in the human brain: 3D (124-ch) EEG power spectrum mapping and source imaging. NeuroImage. 2006;29(4):1080–91.

Chen RC, Huang YH. Acupuncture on experimental epilepsies. Proc Natl Sci Counc Repub China B. 1984;8(1):72–7.

Cheung MJ, Kovacevic N, Fatima Z, et al. [MEG]PLS: a pipeline for MEG data analysis and partial least squares statistics. NeuroImage. 2016;124:181–93.

Chongcheng X, Huansen X, Qingchi R, et al. Electric acupuncture convulsive therapy. Convuls Ther. 1985;1(4):242–51.

Chu NS. A simultaneous comparison of acupuncture needle and insulated needle sphenoidal electrodes for detection of anterior temporal spikes. Clin Electroencephalogr. 1992;23(1):47–51.

Chu NS, Wu CL, Tseng TS, et al. Sphenoidal EEG recording using acupuncture needle electrode in complex partial seizure. Electroencephalogr Clin Neurophysiol. 1991;79(2):119–26.

Cohen D, Cuffin BN, Yunokuchi K, et al. MEG versus EEG localization test using implanted sources in the human brain. Ann Neurol. 1990;28:811–7.

Colbert AP, Cleaver J, Brown KA, et al. Magnets applied to acupuncture points as therapy: a literature review. Acupunct Med. 2008;26(3):160–70.

Ding YH, Gu CY, Shen LR, et al. Effects of acupuncture combined general anesthesia on endorphin and hemodynamics of laparoscopic cholecystectomy patients in the perioperative phase. Zhongguo Zhong Xi Yi Jie He Za Zhi. 2013;33(6):761–5.

Dale AM, Halgren E. Spatiotemporal mapping of brain activity by integration of multiple imaging modalities. Curr Opin Neurobiol. 2001;11(2):202–8.

Dhond RP, Kettner N, Napadow V. Neuroimaging acupuncture effects in the human brain. J Altern Complement Med. 2007a;13(6):603–16.

Dhond RP, Witzel T, Yeh C, et al. Mapping the neural correlates of acupuncture with magnetoencephalography. Baltimore: Society for Acupuncture Research; 2007b.

Florin E, Baillet S. The brain's resting-state activity is shaped by synchronized cross-frequency coupling of neural oscillations. NeuroImage. 2015;111:26–35.

Gamaleia NF, Stadnik V, Rudykh ZM, et al. Experimental validation and the initial experience of the use of intravenous laser irradiation of the blood in oncology. Eksp Onkol. 1988;10(2):60–3.

Gao H, Yan L, Liu B, et al. Clinical study on treatment of senile vascular dementia by acupuncture. J Tradit Chin Med. 2001;21(2):103–9.

Geng Y, Zhang X. EEG EPs analysis of magnetic stimulation on acupoint of Shenmen(HT7). Conf Proc IEEE Eng Med Biol Soc. 2012;2012:5745–8.

George JS, Jackson PS, Ranken DM, et al. Three-dimensional volumetric reconstruction for neuromagnetic source localization. In: Williamson SJ, Hoke M, Stroink G, et al., editors. Advances in biomagnetism. New York: Plenum Press; 1989. p. 737–40.

Goiz-Marquez G, Caballero S, Solis H, et al. Electroencephalographic evaluation of gold wire implants inserted in acupuncture points in dogs with epileptic seizures. Res Vet Sci. 2009;86(1):152–61.

Atwood HL, MacKay WA. Essentials of neurophysiology. Toronto: Decker; 1989.

Haas L. Hans Berger (1873–1941), Richard Caton (1842–1926), and electroencephalography. J Neurol Neurosurg Psychiatry. 2003;74(1):9.

Hari R, Hamalainen M, Ilmoniemi R, et al. MEG versus EEG localization test (Letter to the Editor). Ann Neurol. 1991;30:222–4.

He B, Yang L, Wilke C, et al. Electrophysiological imaging of brain activity and connectivity—challenges and opportunities. IEEE Trans Biomed Eng. 2011;58:1918–31.

He W, Litscher G, Jing XH, et al. Effectiveness of interstitial laser acupuncture depends upon dosage: experimental results from electrocardiographic and electrocorticographic recordings. Evid Based Complement Alternat Med. 2013a;2013:934783.

He W, Litscher G, Wang X, et al. Intravenous laser blood irradiation, interstitial laser acupuncture, and electroacupuncture in an animal experimental setting: preliminary results from heart rate variability and electrocorticographic recordings. Evid Based Complement Alternat Med. 2013b;2013:169249.

Jasper H. Report of committee on methods of clinical exam in EEG. Electroencephalogr Clin Neurophysiol. 1958;10:370–5.

Johannisson T. Correlations between personality traits and specific groups of alpha waves in the human EEG. Peer J. 2016;4:e2245.

Juel J, Liguori S, Liguori A, et al. A new method for sham-controlled acupuncture in experimental visceral pain: a randomized, single-blinded study. Pain Pract. 2016;16(6):669–79.

Kakigi R, Inui K, Tamura Y. Electrophysiological studies on human pain perception. Clin Neurophysiol. 2005;116(4):743–63.

Kaufman L, Schwartz B, Salustri C, et al. Modulation of spontaneous brain activity during mental imagery. J Cogn Neurosci. 1990;2:124–32.

Kim MS, Nam TC. Electroencephalography (EEG) spectral edge frequency for assessing the sedative effect of acupuncture in dogs. J Vet Med Sci. 2006;68(4):409–11.

Kim MS, Soh KS, Nam TC, et al. Evaluation of sedation on electroencephalographic spectral edge frequency 95 in dogs sedated by acupuncture at GV20 or Yintang and sedative combination. Acupunct Electrother Res. 2006;31(3–4):201–12.

Kim MS, Kim HD, Seo HD, et al. The effect of acupuncture at PC-6 on the electroencephalogram and electrocardiogram. Am J Chin Med. 2008;36(3):481–91.

Kim MS, Cho YC, Moon JH, et al. A characteristic estimation of bio-signals for electro-acupuncture stimulations in human subjects. Am J Chin Med. 2009;37(3):505–17.

Kim K, Begus S, Xia H, et al. Multi-channel atomic magnetometer for magnetoencephalography: a configuration study. NeuroImage. 2014;89:143–51.

Korochkin IM, Ioseliani DG, Berkinbaev SF, et al. Treatment of acute myocardial infarction by intravenous irradiation of the blood using helium-neon laser. Sov Med. 1988;4:34–8.

Kotini A, Anninos P. Alpha, delta and theta rhythms in a neural net model. Comparison with MEG data. J Theor Biol. 2016;388:11–4.

Lappe C, Lappe M, Pantev C. Differential processing of melodic, rhythmic and simple tone deviations in musicians: an MEG study. NeuroImage. 2016;124:898–905.

Lee FS, Chang TA, Wu A. Pain induced by intensive light beam pulse stimulation of acupuncture point GB34 of lower extremities and its associated changes in EEG's. Acupunct Electrother Res. 2011;36(3–4):275–86.

Lin FH, Witzel T, Hamalainen MS, et al. Spectral spatiotemporal imaging of cortical oscillations and interactions in the human brain. NeuroImage. 2004;23:582–95.

Lina JM, Chowdhury R, Lemay E, et al. Wavelet-based localization of oscillatory sources from magnetoencephalography data. IEEE Trans Biomed Eng. 2014;61:2350–64.

Litscher G, Wang L, Wiesner-Zechmeister M. Specific effects of laserpuncture on the cerebral circulation. Lasers Med Sci. 2000;15(1):57–62.

Litscher G. Effects of acupressure, manual acupuncture and Laserneedle acupuncture on EEG bispectral index and spectral edge frequency in healthy volunteers. Eur J Anaesthesiol. 2004;21(1):13–9.

Liu AK, Dale AM, Belliveau JW. Monte Carlo simulation studies of EEG and MEG localization accuracy. Hum Brain Mapp. 2002;16:47–62.

Liu X, Wang J, Wang B, et al. Effect of transcutaneous acupoint electrical stimulation on propofol sedation: an electroencephalogram analysis of patients undergoing pituitary adenomas resection. BMC Complement Altern Med. 2016;16:33.

Logothetis NK, Pauls J, Augath M, et al. Neurophysiological investigation of the basis of the fMRI signal. Nature. 2001;412:150–7.

Lutkenhoner B. Current Dipole Localization with an ideal magnetometer system. IEEE Trans Biomed Eng. 1996;43:1049–61.

Lutkenhoner B. Some statistical aspects of magnetoencephalography. In: Moore M, editor. Spatial statistics: methodological aspects and applications. New York: Springer; 2001. p. 213–45.

Lutkenhoner B. Magnetoencephalography and its Achilles' heel. J Physiol Paris. 2003;97(4–6): 641–58.

Mantini D, Penna DS, Marzetti L, et al. A signal-processing pipeline for magnetoencephalography resting-state networks. Brain Connect. 2011;1(1):49–59.

Mantini D, Franciotti R, Romani GL, et al. Improving MEG source localizations: an automated method for complete artifact removal based on independent component analysis. NeuroImage. 2008;40:160–73.

Menninghaus E, Lutkenhoner B. How silent are deep and radial sources in neuromagnetic measurements? In: Baumgartner C, Deecke L, Stroink G, et al., editors. Biomagnetism: fundamental research and clinical applications. New York: Pergamon Press; 1995. p. 352–6.

Iber C, Ancoli-Israel S, Chesson AL Jr, et al. The AASM manual for the scoring of sleep and associated events: rules, terminology and technical specifications. Westchester: American Academy of Sleep Medicine; 2007.

Miozzo M, Pulvermuller F, Hauk O. Early parallel activation of semantics and phonology in picture naming: evidence from a multiple linear regression MEG study. Cereb Cortex. 2014;25:3343–55.

Nayak S, Wenstone R, Jones A, et al. Surface electrostimulation of acupuncture points for sedation of critically ill patients in the intensive care unit—a pilot study. Acupunct Med. 2008;26(1):1–7.

Orrison WW Jr. Magnetic source imaging in stereotactic and functional neurosurgery. Stereotact Funct Neurosurg. 1999;72(2–4):89–94.

Pei X, Wang J, Deng B, et al. WLPVG approach to the analysis of EEG-based functional brain network under manual acupuncture. Cogn Neurodyn. 2014;8(5):417–28.

Oostenveld R, Praamstra P. The five percent electrode system for high-resolution EEG and ERP measurements. Clin Neurophysiol. 2001;112(4):713–9.

Silva JG, Santana CG, Inocencio KR, et al. Electrocortical analysis of patients with intercostobrachial pain treated with TENS after breast cancer surgery. J Phys Ther Sci. 2014;26(3):349–53.

Siebenhuhner F, Weiss SA, Coppola R, et al. Intra- and inter-frequency brain network structure in health and schizophrenia. PLoS One. 2013;8(8):e72351.

Stokes MG, Wolff MJ, Spaak E. Decoding rich spatial information with high temporal resolution. Trends Cogn Sci. 2015;19(11):636–8.

Supek S, Aine CJ. Simulation studies of multiple dipole neuromagnetic source localization: model order and limits of source resolution. IEEE Trans Biomed Eng. 1993;40(6):529–40.

Supek S, Aine CJ. Spatio-temporal modeling of neuromagnetic data: I. multi-source location versus time-course estimation accuracy. Hum Brain Mapp. 1997;5(3):139–53.

Tan S, Roth BJ, Wikswo JP. The magnetic field of cortical current sources: the application of a spatial filtering model to the forward and inverse problems. Electroencephalogr Clin Neurophysiol. 1990;76(1):73–85.

Taulu S, Kaiola M, Simola J. The signal space separation method. Physics. 2012;1270(9):32–37.

Teplan M. Fundamentals of EEG measurement. Meas Sci Rev. 2002;2(2):1–11.

Wang B, Tang J, White PF, et al. Effect of the intensity of transcutaneous acupoint electrical stimulation on the postoperative analgesic requirement. Anesth Analg. 1997;85(2):406–13.

Wang H, Xie Y, Zhang Q, et al. Transcutaneous electric acupoint stimulation reduces intraoperative remifentanil consumption and alleviates postoperative side-effects in patients undergoing sinusotomy: a prospective, randomized, placebo-controlled trial. Br J Anaesth. 2014;112(6):1075–82.

Weber M. Interstitial and intraarticular laser therapy as an attractive new option for the treatment of spinal cord diseases and chronic joint arthroses. Schmerz & Akupunktur. 2011;2:2–4.

Wikswo JP, Roth BJ. Magnetic determination of the spatial extent of a single cortical current source: a theoretical analysis. Electroencephalogr Clin Neurophysiol. 1988;69(3):266–76.

Williamson S. MEG versus EEG localization test (Letter to the Editor). Ann Neurol. 1991;30(2):222–4.

Yi PL, Tsai CH, Lin JG, et al. Effects of electroacupuncture at 'Anmian (Extra)' acupoints on sleep activities in rats: the implication of the caud al nucleus tractus solitarius. J Biomed Sci. 2004;11(5):579–90.

Yi PL, Lu CY, Jou SB, et al. Low-frequency electroacupuncture suppresses focal epilepsy and improves epilepsy-induced sleep disruptions. J Biomed Sci. 2015;22(1):1–12.

Yi G, Wang J, Bian H, et al. Multi-scale order recurrence quantification analysis of EEG signals evoked by manual acupuncture in healthy subjects. Cogn Neurodyn. 2013;7(1):79–88.

Yin CS, Park HJ, Kim SY, et al. Electroencephalogram changes according to the subjective acupuncture sensation. Neurol Res. 2010;32(Suppl 1):31–6.

You Y, Bai L, Dai R, et al. Acupuncture induces divergent alterations of functional connectivity within conventional frequency bands: evidence from MEG recordings. PLoS One. 2012;7(11):e49250.

You Y, Bai L, Dai R, et al. Altered hub configurations within default mode network following acupuncture at ST36: a multimodal investigation combining fMRI and MEG. PLoS One. 2013;8(5):e64509.

Yu H, Xu G, Yang R, et al. Somatosensory-evoked potentials and cortical activities evoked by magnetic stimulation on acupoint in human. Conf Proc IEEE Eng Med Biol Soc. 2009;2009:3445–8.

Prospects of Acupuncture Research in the Future

5

Wei Qin, Lingmin Jin, and Jie Tian

5.1 Introduction

In the previous chapters, we have systematically introduced what is currently known about acupuncture, its therapeutic effects, and its neurological substrates based on neuroimaging studies. Neuroimaging techniques including functional magnetic resonance imaging (fMRI), electroencephalography (EEG), and magnetoencephalography (MEG) have been used to assess changes in brain activity in response to external acupuncture stimulation in a variety of contexts. These changes are represented in a number of dynamic brain networks with various time-varied activation patterns that are presumed to reflect specific effects of acupuncture. Accordingly, perspectives from neuroscience research suggest that the treatment effects of acupuncture are at least in part mediated by functional alterations in brain network activity.

In acupuncture fMRI studies, acupuncture stimulation tasks were initially designed to study specific brain responses to stimulation (Wu et al. 2002; Yoo et al. 2004). Over time, resting-state alterations in activity and specifically intrinsic information about the macroscale spatiotemporal organization of the brain were investigated with respect to acupuncture (Liu et al. 2009; Jiang et al. 2012; Wang et al. 2014). Using functional connectivity analyses, a number of resting-state brain networks (intrinsic connectivity networks, ICNs) have been recognized for their potential involvement in therapeutic acupuncture effects. These ICNs include the default mode network (Greicius et al. 2003; Baliki et al. 2008), motor network (Biswal et al. 1995), ventral and dorsal attention networks (Ptak 2012; Viviani 2013), and salience network (Seeley et al. 2007). In recent years, a more detailed parcellation

W. Qin • L. Jin
School of Life Sciences and Technology, Xidian University, Xi'an, China

J. Tian (✉)
CAS Key Laboratory of Molecular Imaging, Institute of Automation, Beijing, China
e-mail: jie.tian@ia.ac.cn

© Springer Nature Singapore Pte Ltd. 2018

J. Tian (ed.), *Multi-Modality Neuroimaging Study on Neurobiological Mechanisms of Acupuncture*, DOI 10.1007/978-981-10-4914-9_5

has facilitated further insights about connectivity among these large-scale multiple brain networks (Calhoun et al. 2008; Calhoun and Adali 2012). Accordingly, acupuncture studies have recently begun to evaluate modulatory effects on these internetwork connections (Liang et al. 2014; Chen et al. 2015; Jia et al. 2015).

5.2 Dynamic Functional Network Connectivity Research

Functional connections between brain areas are gradually recognized as dynamic, where the connections may transiently appear with time (Allen et al. 2014). A new approach defined as dynamic functional network connectivity (d-FNC) is applied to divide resting-state fMRI (rsfMRI) images into series of continuous "sliding windows" to evaluate the dynamic functional connections. These sliding windows can offer a much more accurate characterization of dynamic brain function on the order of seconds rather than minutes (Allen et al. 2014; Nomi et al. 2016).

5.2.1 Limitations of Resting-State Functional Connectivity Analysis

In the last decade, assessments of functional connectivity across the duration of a scan or task have become increasingly popular. These assessments are most commonly conducted by correlating regional changes in activity in an approach known as the static functional network connectivity (s-FNC) approach. However, there are some problems with this approach; firstly, spontaneous fluctuations which can emerge over timescales spanning from milliseconds to dozens of minutes are a trait of signal recordings. Yet, intrinsic brain network researches based on rsfMRI have mainly ignored the temporal variability of signal recordings (Allen et al. 2014). Most current approaches implicitly hypothesize that the relationships remain unchanged throughout the length of the record. While this assumption is convenient in that it limits the complexity of whole-brain analysis, it also regrettably expresses a gross oversimplification. That is, s-FNC approaches may obscure unique modes of dynamic brain activity. Secondly, because mental activity is unconstrained during the resting state, dynamic state potentially becomes more prominent (compared to the active state). It is demonstrated that subjects are freely concerned with several types of psychological activity in resting state. The predominant type of activity (e.g., imagery or inner language) influences the whole-brain functional connectivity and modular organization (Allen et al. 2014). Given that resting-state mental activity is not controlled in this aspect, study generalizability and comparability may be compromised.

5.2.2 Necessity of Dynamic Research

A number of inconsistencies have been noted between studies employing the s-FNC approach (Fornito et al. 2012; Keilholz et al. 2013; Allen et al. 2014). For example, in the context of schizophrenia research, research has offered conflicting reports of hyperconnectivity and hypoconnectivity between the same brain regions (Fornito et al. 2012). Although this could be in part due to differences in disease subtypes or symptoms, another reasonable explanation is that static connectivity obtained by averaging whole time courses fails to distinguish temporal variations in network connectivity. Previous studies on time-varying characteristic of brain functional connection consider that temporal variations are reflections of the significative dynamic properties (Keilholz et al. 2013; Thompson et al. 2013, 2014). In particular, highly structured and quasi-stable connection pattern which reoccurred over time could be evaluated as "connectivity states" (Allen et al. 2014).

5.2.3 Dynamic Research Application

On the above premise, a growing number of studies have focused on dynamic variations in functional connectivity (Shen et al. 2015; Yu et al. 2015; Nomi et al. 2016; Yoo et al. 2016). The findings of these studies have provided new insights into biomarkers of mental disorders and functional impairments in brain performance. In this section, we will examine two dynamic research studies in order to provide a clearer perspective of what dynamic research can offer to the field of acupuncture neuroimaging.

5.2.3.1 A Dynamic Variety Analysis of Whole-Brain Functional Connectivity

Yu and colleagues developed an important framework for assessing dynamic properties of timing-varying functional connectivity in resting fMRI data and applied this framework to evaluate differences between schizophrenia patients (SZs) and health control subjects (HCs) (Yu et al. 2015). In this study, a total of 82 SZs and 82 age- and gender-matched HCs were involved. The data preprocessing of all 164 participants was performed using the SPM8 toolbox (http://www.fsl.ion.ucl.ac.uk/spm), and a spatial group independent component analysis (ICA) was implemented using the GIFT software package (http://mialab.mrn.org/software/gift). All the data were then decomposed into 100 aggregate components, from which 48 proper independent components (ICs) were chosen as ICNs. Time courses for each of the 48 ICs underwent additional post-processing, including detrending, multiple regression, detected outliers removing, and band-pass filtering. Then, each subject's s-FNC was computed, and pairwise correlations were defined between ICN time courses. Compared to HCs, SZs exhibited irregular intrinsic network connectivity (Fig. 5.1).

A dynamic connectivity analysis of each participant was completed by combining a sliding time window approach (with a width of $L = 20$ repetition time (TR) in 1-TR steps) with a graph theory approach. A sliding time window approach was used to obtain dynamic time courses so that ICN correlations could be computed during each dynamic time course. Accordingly, the authors were able to examine all d-FNCs for each subject. Graph theory was then applied to compute connectivity strengths, clustering coefficients, and global

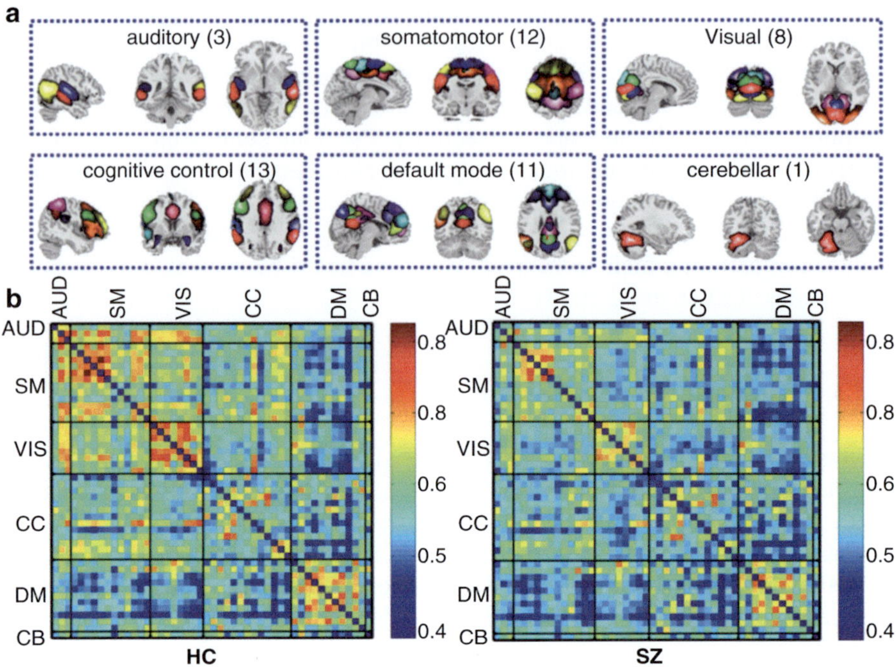

Fig. 5.1 Spatial maps of 48 intrinsic connectivity networks (**a**) and the stationary functional connectivity (similarity S matrix); (**b**) between them in healthy control subjects (HC) and schizophrenia patients (SZ) (Reprint with permission from Yu et al. 2015). Intrinsic connectivity networks are divided into groups and arranged based on their anatomical and functional properties. Functional connectivity was averaged over all subjects in each group. *AUD* auditory, *CB* cerebellar, *CC* cognitive control, *DM* default mode, *SM* somatomotor, *VIS* visual

efficiencies for d-FNCs using the brain connectivity toolbox (http://www.brain-connectivity-toolbox.net/; BCT). To determine relationships among d-FNCs, the authors applied first- and second-level analyses: first, the modularity algorithm of Newman (2006) was applied to the window correlation metrics of each subject, averaging the d-FNC within the same module, to yield a total of 554 states (276 states in HCs and 278 states in SZs). Second, the algorithm was applied to all 554 states to produce one final state (Fig. 5.2).

Of note, only one connectivity state is identified by the second-level analysis. In this example, a total of 271 first-level connectivity states (155 states in 75 HCs and 116 states in 67 SZs) that were highly associated with one another were averaged into the second-level state. Compared with HCs, SZs exhibited fewer first-level connectivity states that were subsequently associated with the

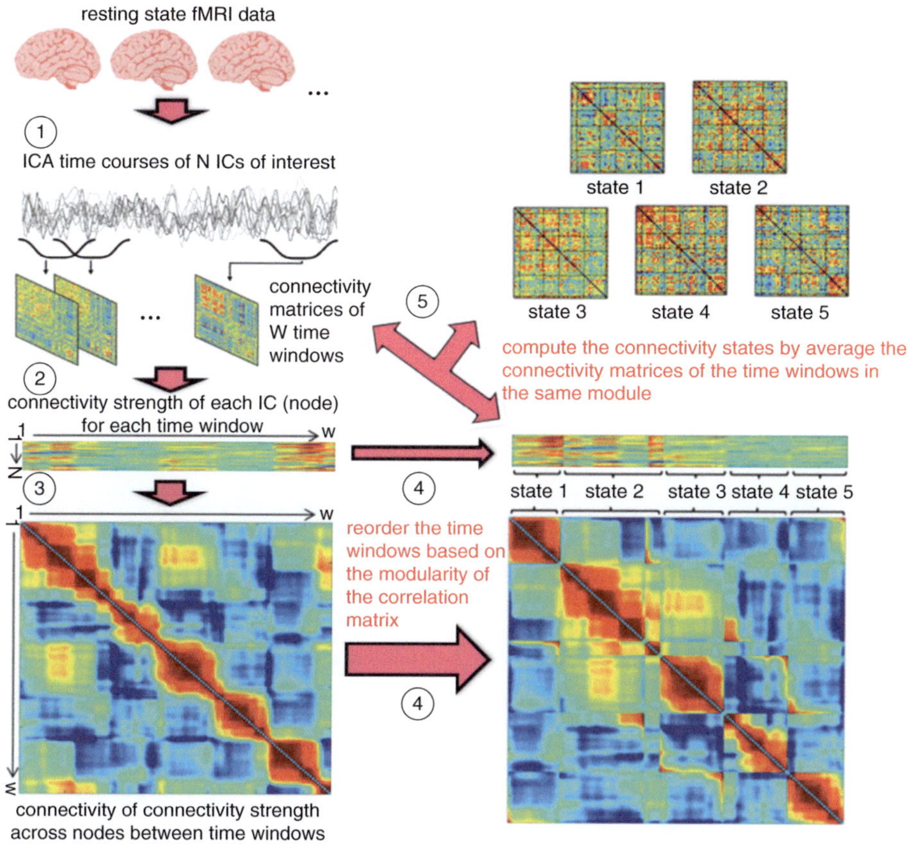

Fig. 5.2 Flowchart of the algorithmic pipeline for the first-level connectivity state analysis (Reprint with permission from Yu et al. 2015)

second-level connectivity state. Moreover, the 155 first-level states in HCs showed higher ($P < 0.01$, two-sample t-tests of the means and permutation tests of medians) graph metrics than the 116 first-level states in SZs (Fig. 5.3). It is noteworthy that, visually, the pattern of the second-level connectivity state in Fig. 5.3 resembles the stationary connectivity pattern shown in Fig. 5.1.

The above work reveals a new way to discover and explore the dynamic properties of network functional connectivity in the context of the healthy brain and neurological disease. An improved understanding of how these properties are altered in various disease states will improve the utility of dynamic connectivity research for understanding disease pathology and therapeutic opportunities in neurological research.

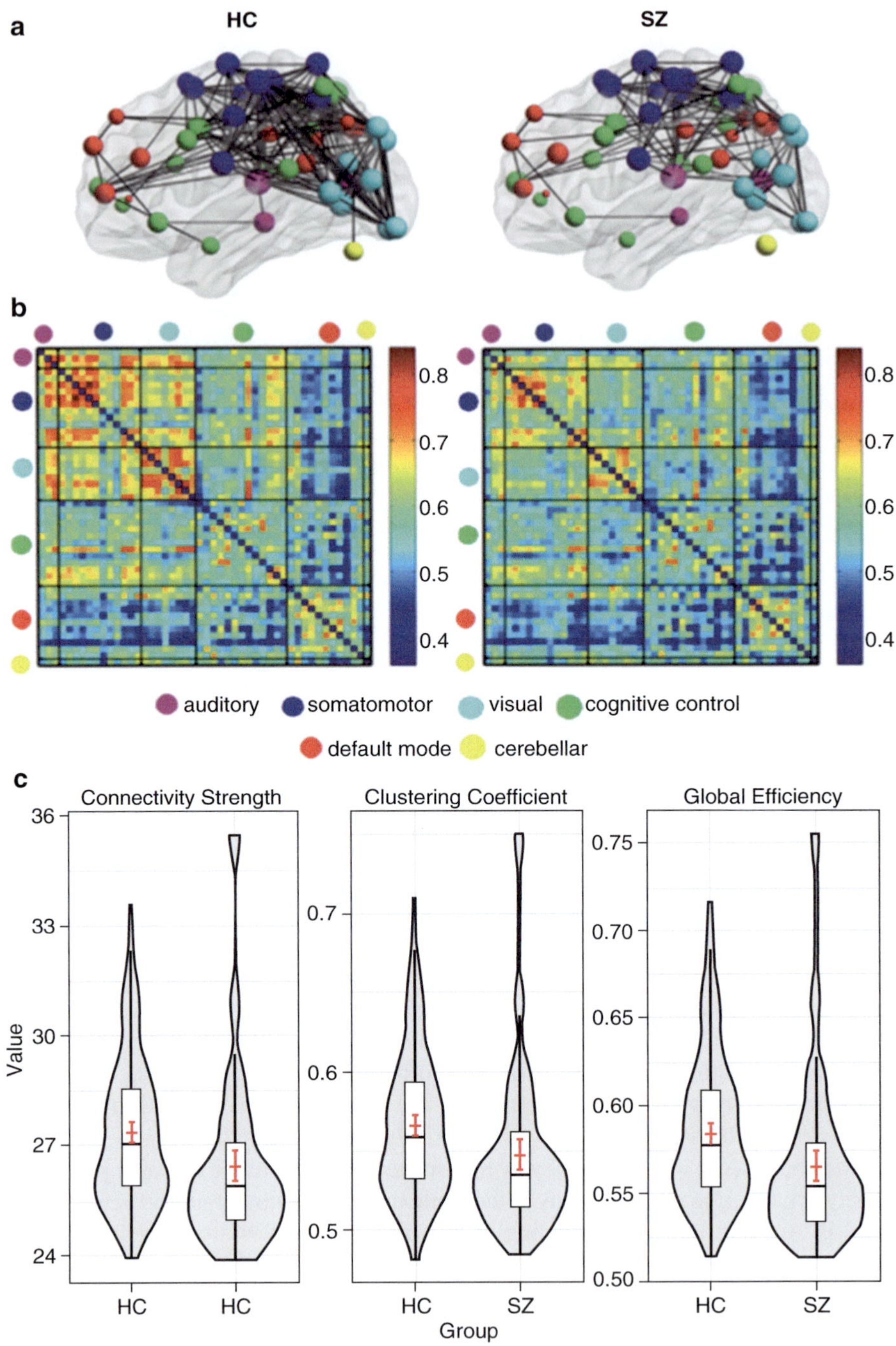

Fig. 5.3 Schematic of the connectivity patterns (Reprint with permission from Yu et al. 2015). (**a**) node size represents nodal connectivity strength (edge threshold = 0.65); (**b**) structures and distribution of graph metrics (**c**) (mean and bootstrapped 95% confidence intervals are in *red*; box plots and smoothed density histograms are also shown) for the first-level connectivity states related to the second-level connectivity state in healthy control subjects (HC, 155 states) and schizophrenia patients (SZ, 116 states), respectively

5.2.3.2 A Dynamic Variety Analysis of Specific Brain Region Functional Connectivity

In the above study, we learned that a dynamic analysis approach can be used to identify neural biomarkers of mental illness. Next, we will introduce a different approach that was used by Nomi and colleagues to analyze the dynamic properties of a specific brain region, the insula (Nomi et al. 2016).

Nomi and colleagues performed an analysis on resting-state fMRI scan data from 31 healthy adult subjects (ages 18–40 years) downloaded from the Nathan Kline Institute database. Data preprocessing, group ICA, and post-processing were performed in a manner similar to that in the previously discussed study by Yu et al. (Fig. 5.4); however, this work used the DPARSF-A toolbox (http://rfmri.org/DPARSF) for data preprocessing, selected 52 no-noise ICs, and identified four of them as belonging to the insular cortex (the dorsal, ventral, posterior, and middle insula).

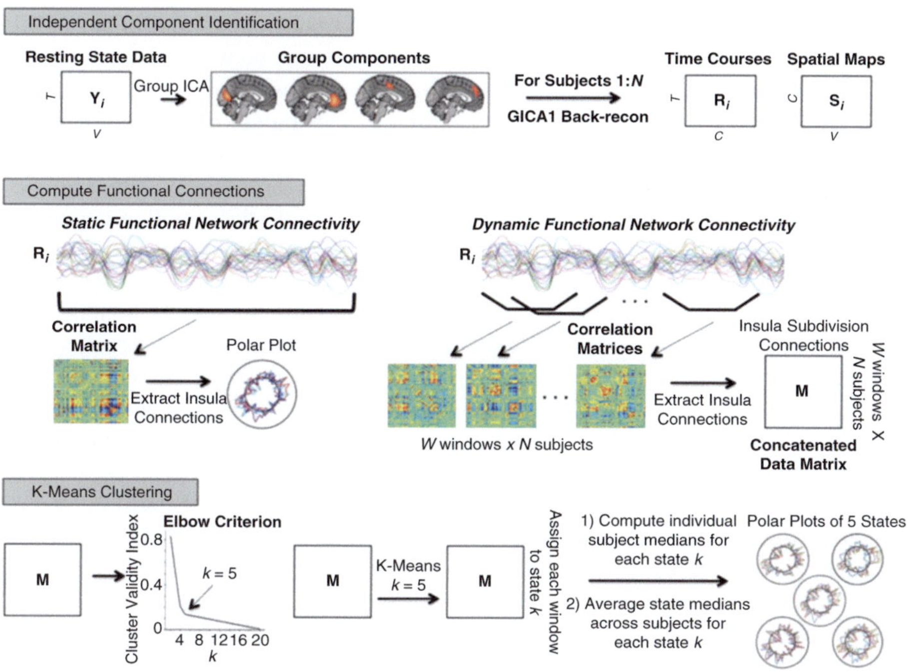

Fig. 5.4 Schematic of the dynamic variety analysis preprocessing performed by Nomi et al. (Reprint with permission from Nomi et al. 2016). (**a**) A high-model group independent component analysis (ICA; 100 components) was used to create a functional parcellation of the brain, resulting in 52 non-noise components. (**b**) Subject-specific time courses from the group ICA were then used to compute functional connections. The static analysis entailed computing correlations over the whole duration of the resting state. The dynamic analysis included acquiring correlation matrices of each subject by employing 45-s tapered-sliding windows (in 1-TR steps) and extracting the connections between each insular subdivision and all other ICS. (**c**) A concatenated data matrix from step B received *k*-means clustering using values 2–20 that identified the optimal *k* as 5 using the elbow criterion; the value of $k = 5$ then assigned each window to dynamic state *k* regardless of subject assignment. Finally subject-specific medians for each state *k* were calculated and averaged together to produce a total of five final dynamic insular states

S-FNCs were computed for each subject, and one-sample t-tests were conducted to identify significant positive connectivities between insular subdivisions and other ICs. In order to assess differences in connectivity strength between insular subdivisions and other ICs, t-tests were conducted on the functional connectivity values. Dynamic functional connectivity was computed in the same way as that described in Yu et al.; however, instead of using graph theory to cluster all d-FNCs, the K-means algorithm was used to partition data into a set of separate clusters, producing final five dynamic insula connectivity states. State 3 was the most frequent occurring insular state (38%; $n = 31$) and was analogous to the s-FNC finding in that unique functional profiles for each insular subdivision could be observed, but State 3 was much smaller in magnitude than s-FNC. State 1 (24%; $n = 31$), State 4 (13%; $n = 26$), and State 5 (20%; $n = 30$) were moderately represented. Finally, State 2 (5%; $n = 59$) was the most infrequent insular state. One-sample t-tests were used to evaluate insular connectivity states in a manner similar to that used for s-FNC data.

Figure 5.5 summarizes the significant positive connections found in the s-FNC analysis. In the static condition, the positive connections between insular subdivisions and other ICs displayed as follows: the connections between the dorsal anterior insula and frontal areas, the connections of the middle and posterior insula with sensorimotor areas, and the connections between ventral insula and ICs representing affective subcortical areas including the nucleus accumbens, hippocampus, and amygdala. These connections are consistent with the emotion-cognition-interoception framework of insular subdivision function (Cauda et al. 2011).

Also depicted in Fig. 5.5 are positive correlations between insular subdivisions and other ICs in each dynamic state. State 3 was similar to the s-FNC. In State 1, all four insular subdivisions showed connections with sensorimotor, temporal, visual, central executive network, and salience network ICs. In addition, the middle insula also exhibited connections with the cerebellum, while the posterior insula was the only region that did not have connections with frontal areas. The results suggest that all the insula subdivisions keep in step with the frontal cortex to process and integrate sensorimotor and visual information in State 1. In State 2, only the dorsal anterior insula appeared connections with subcortical ICs and DMN, while the medial, posterior, and ventral insula showed connectivity with temporal, sensorimotor, and salience network ICs. This suggests that in State 2, the medial, posterior, and ventral subdivisions of the insula work together to coordinate sensorimotor and temporal information, while the dorsal insula works independently to coordinate communication between subcortical areas and the DMN.

Figure 5.6 shows a polar plot of s-FNC correlations for the four subdivisions of the insula. Significant differences in connection strengths between each subdivision with other ICs are identified by an asterisk placed along the radiating axis. The dorsal anterior insula showed stronger connections with frontal brain areas than all other insula subdivisions, particularly with the frontal pole. By contrast, the ventral insula showed significantly stronger connections with ICs representing the nucleus accumbens, hippocampus, and amygdala. These findings are in accordance with the findings of previous studies (Cauda et al. 2011, 2012).

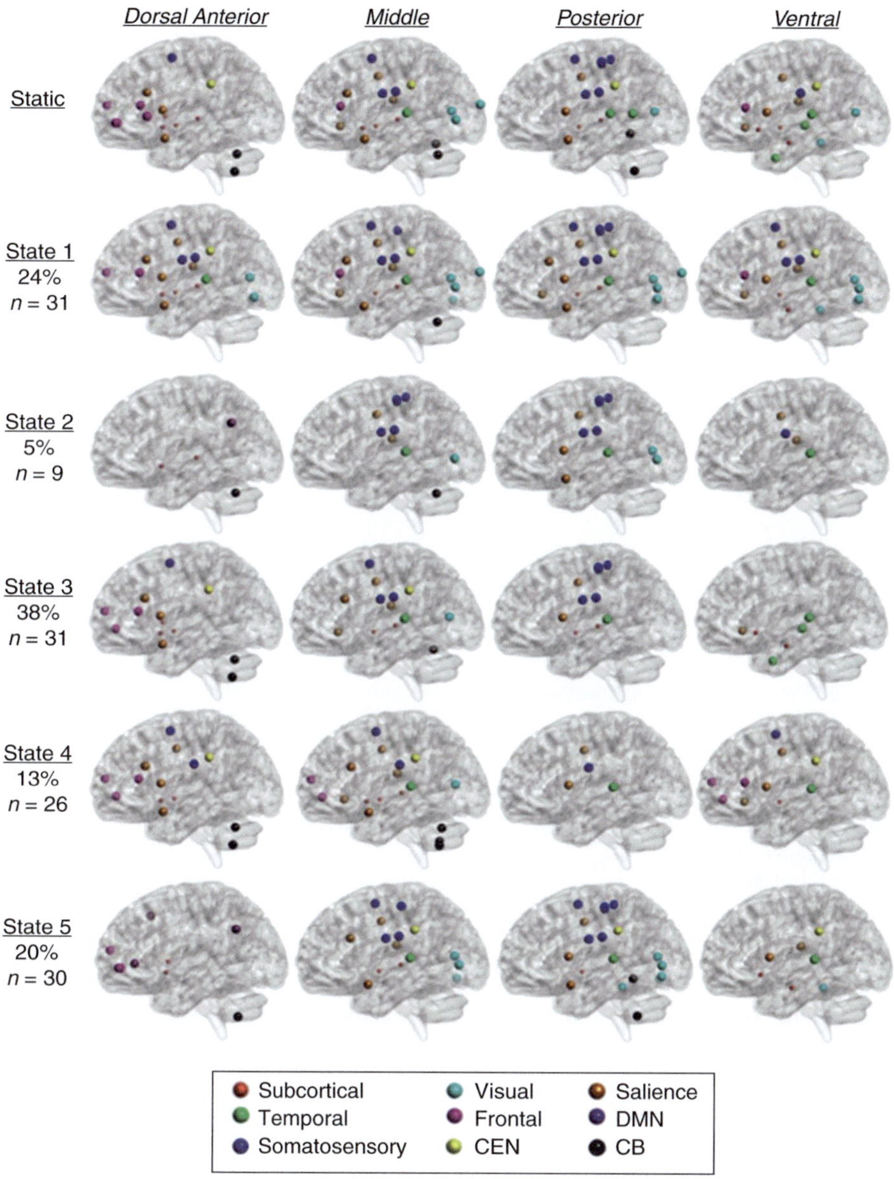

Fig. 5.5 Plots of significant positive connections between insular subdivisions and other ICs (Reprint with permission from Nomi et al. 2016). *CB* cerebellum, *CEN* central executive network, *DMN* default mode network

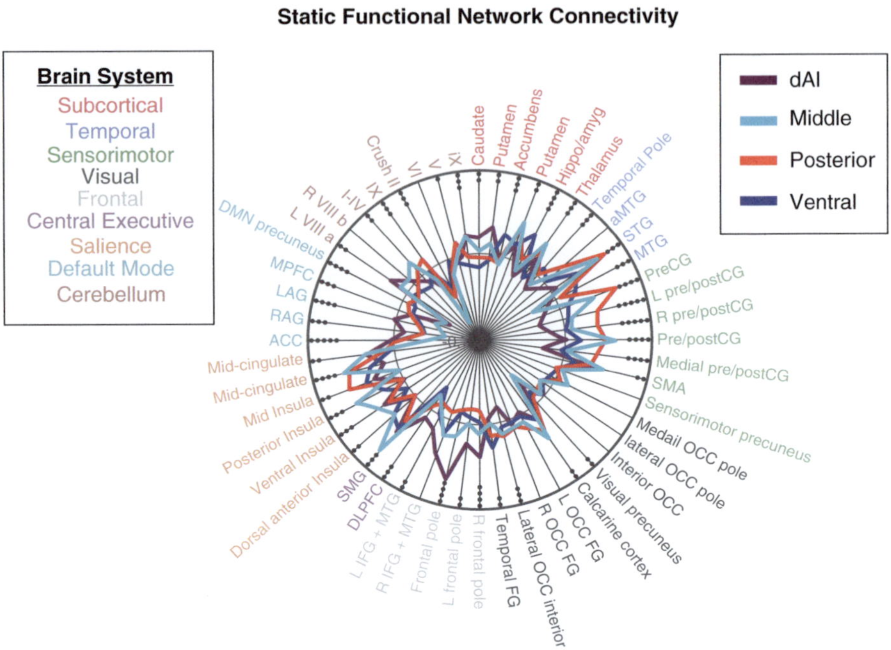

Fig. 5.6 Polar plot displaying functional connections between insular subdivisions and ICs in the static functional connectivity analysis (Reprint with permission from Nomi et al. 2016). *dAI* dorsal anterior insula, *STG* superior temporal gyrus, *MTG* medial temporal gyrus, *IFG* inferior frontal gyrus, *CG* central gyrus, *SMA* supplementary motor area, *OCC* occipital, *CC* calcarine cortex, *FG* fusiform gyrus, *ACC* anterior cingulate cortex, *OBF* orbitofrontal cortex, *DLPFC* dorsal lateral prefrontal cortex, *AG* angular gyrus, *MPFC* medial prefrontal cortex, *DMN* default mode network, *SMG* supramarginal gyrus

Figure 5.7 shows a similar polar plot to that in Fig. 5.6, but instead represents functional connections in each of the five dynamic states. State 1 had 41 significant differences across the insular subdivisions, State 2 had 33, State 3 had 77, State 4 had 61, and State 5 had 113. States with fewer significant changes accordingly represent that insular subdivisions exhibited more common connections to various ICs (convergence across subdivision connections), while states with more changes mean that insular subdivisions exhibited more individual connectivity profiles with various ICs (divergence across connections).

These results highlight the way in which functional dynamics can be captured by a d-FNC approach based on the s-FNC mark. In this particular study, a d-FNC approach revealed the functional flexibility of the insula over time.

In summary, research on the temporal properties of functional connectivity can reveal complex flexibility in functional coordination among distinct brain networks and improve our understanding of behavioral shifts and adaptive processes in the human brain. These techniques have significant utility for the study of acupuncture, especially given the important and diverse time-dependent alterations in brain activity associated with acupuncture therapy.

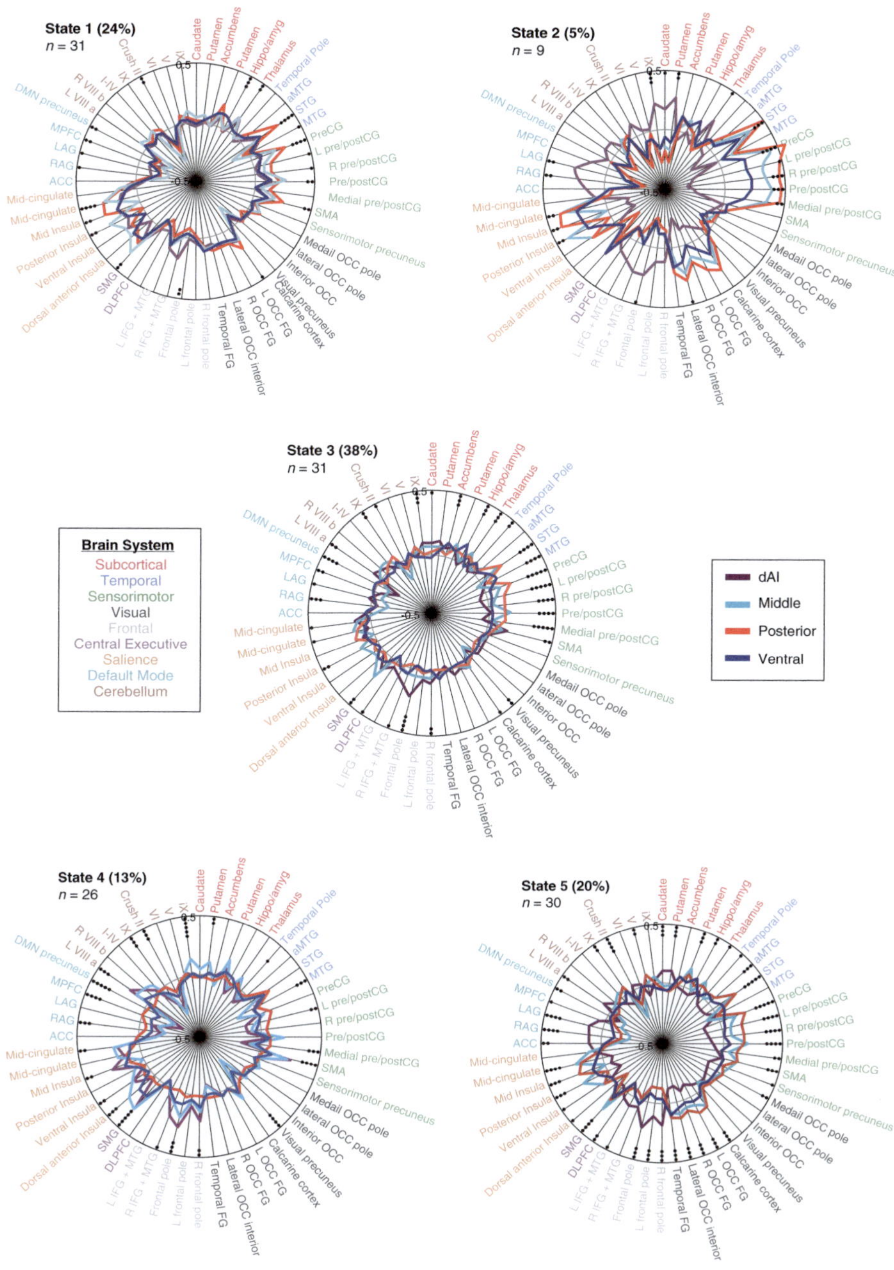

Fig. 5.7 Polar plots representing functional connections between insular subdivisions and ICs in the whole insula dynamic functional connectivity analysis (Reprint with permission from Nomi et al. 2016). *dAI* dorsal anterior insula, *STG* superior temporal gyrus, *MTG* medial temporal gyrus, *IFG* inferior frontal gyrus, *CG* central gyrus, *SMA* supplementary motor area, *OCC* occipital, *CC* calcarine cortex, *FG* fusiform gyrus, *ACC* anterior cingulate cortex, *OBF* orbitofrontal cortex, *DLPFC* dorsal lateral prefrontal cortex, *AG* angular gyrus, *MPFC* medial prefrontal cortex, *DMN* default mode network, *SMG* supramarginal gyrus

5.3 A Framework for Future fMRI Studies of Acupuncture

As described in previous chapters, the progress of acupuncture research has been slowed by inappropriate study design, poor statistical power, and a number of methodological issues resulting in study heterogeneity. Here, we propose several suggestions for the future conduct of acupuncture fMRI research.

5.3.1 Study Populations

In 2002, the World Health Organization Consultation on Acupuncture reviewed data from controlled clinical trials of acupuncture and identified nearly 100 disease states and disorders for which acupuncture had potential or demonstrated efficacy (WHO 2002). To study the mechanisms of acupuncture efficacy, we recommend that future studies focus on patients within indications for acupuncture therapy rather than healthy subjects. There are several important barriers to understanding the central mechanisms of acupuncture; of these, a better understanding of immediate and persistent responses to acupuncture and the key pathological mechanisms affected by acupuncture are highly important and can be informed by comparing differences between patient and healthy control subject responses to stimulation at the same acupoints.

5.3.2 Analytical Methodology

The use of appropriate data-driven methods for the analysis of fMRI studies is highly important for providing accurate characterizations of neural responses to acupuncture. Furthermore, with the development of imaging research methodology, diverse analysis approaches which like functional connectivity (Qin et al. 2008; Deng et al. 2016b; Shi et al. 2016), independent component analysis (Zhang et al. 2009; Liu et al. 2010), graph theoretic analysis (Bai et al. 2009), multi-voxel pattern analysis (Li et al. 2010), multivariate Granger causality analysis (Zhong et al. 2012), and regional homogeneity (Deng et al. 2016a) have become available for use to satisfy different research objectives of acupuncture studies. The analysis of dynamic functional network connectivity described in this chapter is considered to be one of the most objective and accurate analysis methods currently available. The monitoring of brain network flexibility has the potential to reveal dynamic responses evoked by acupuncture and should thus be applied in future acupuncture fMRI studies.

5.3.3 Research Instruments

As outlined in the previous chapters, a variety of imaging instruments have been employed in acupuncture studies, such as fMRI, EEG, MEG, and positron emission tomography. Every tool has specific advantages; for example, fMRI provides high spatial resolution, while EEG and MEG provide high temporal resolution. However, most acupuncture studies to date have only analyzed and reported data from a single imaging modality. Multimodal fusion imaging can provide high spatiotemporal resolution and integrate larger amounts of information to provide more robust and detailed hypotheses about the central mechanisms of acupuncture. Future acupuncture studies should take advantage of multimodal fusion imaging as a highly useful and attractive research tool.

5.4 Summary

Nearly two decades have elapsed since the first article of acupuncture fMRI research was published. Since then, the field of acupuncture neuroimaging has exploded, yielding a number of achievements and additional research questions. To encourage the conduct of future high-quality acupuncture neuroimaging studies, we have summarized the tools and studies available to acupuncture research and proposed that additional studies focus enrolling patients with acupuncture indications, use multimodal fusion imaging techniques to collect imaging data, and carefully adopt suitable analysis approaches for the processing of the resultant data.

References

Allen EA, Damaraju E, Plis SM, et al. Tracking whole-brain connectivity dynamics in the resting state. Cereb Cortex. 2014;24(3):663–76.

Bai L, Qin W, Tian J, et al. Detection of dynamic brain networks modulated by acupuncture using a graph theory model. Prog Nat Sci. 2009;19(7):827–35.

Baliki MN, Geha PY, Apkarian AV, et al. Beyond feeling: chronic pain hurts the brain, disrupting the default-mode network dynamics. J Neurosci. 2008;28(6):1398–403.

Biswal B, Yetkin FZ, Haughton VM, et al. Functional connectivity in the motor cortex of resting human brain using echo-planar MRI. Magn Reson Med. 1995;34(4):537–41.

Cauda F, D'Agata F, Sacco K, et al. Functional connectivity of the insula in the resting brain. NeuroImage. 2011;55:8–23.

Cauda F, Costa T, Torta DM, et al. Meta-analytic clustering of the insular cortex: characterizing the meta-analytic connectivity of the insula when involved in active tasks. NeuroImage. 2012;62:343–55.

Calhoun VD, Adali T. Multisubject independent component analysis of fMRI: a decade of intrinsic networks, default mode, and neurodiagnostic discovery. IEEE Rev Biomed Eng. 2012;5:60–73.

Calhoun VD, Kiehl KA, Pearlson GD. Modulation of temporally coherent brain networks estimated using ICA at rest and during cognitive tasks. Hum Brain Mapp. 2008;29(7):828–38.

Chen X, Zhang H, Zou Y. A functional magnetic resonance imaging study on the effect of acupuncture at GB34 (Yanglingquan) on motor-related network in hemiplegic patients. Brain Res. 2015;1601:64–72.

Deng D, Duan G, Liao H, et al. Changes in regional brain homogeneity induced by electro-acupuncture stimulation at the baihui acupoint in healthy subjects: a functional magnetic resonance imaging study. J Altern Complement Med. 2016a;22(10):794–9.

Deng D, Liao H, Duan G, et al. Modulation of the default mode network in first-episode, drug-naive major depressive disorder via acupuncture at Baihui (GV20) acupoint. Front Hum Neurosci. 2016b;10:230.

Fornito A, Zalesky A, Pantelis C, et al. Schizophrenia, neuroimaging and connectomics. NeuroImage. 2012;62(4):2296–314.

Greicius MD, Krasnow B, Reiss AL, et al. Functional connectivity in the resting brain: a network analysis of the default mode hypothesis. Proc Natl Acad Sci U S A. 2003;100(1):253–8.

Jia B, Liu Z, Min B, et al. The effects of acupuncture at real or sham acupoints on the intrinsic brain activity in mild cognitive impairment patients. Evid Based Complement Alternat Med. 2015;2015:529675.

Jiang Y, Hao Y, Zhang Y, et al. Thirty minute transcutaneous electric acupoint stimulation modulates resting state brain activities: a perfusion and BOLD fMRI study. Brain Res. 2012;1457:13–25.

Keilholz SD, Magnuson ME, Pan WJ, et al. Dynamic properties of functional connectivity in the rodent. Brain Connect. 2013;3(1):31–40.

Li L, Qin W, Bai L, et al. Exploring vision-related acupuncture point specificity with multivoxel pattern analysis. Magn Reson Imaging. 2010;28(3):380–7.

Liang P, Wang Z, Qian T, et al. Acupuncture stimulation of Taichong (Liv3) and Hegu (LI4) modulates the default mode network activity in Alzheimer's disease. Am J Alzheimers Dis Other Demen. 2014;29(8):739–48.

Liu P, Zhang Y, Zhou G, et al. Partial correlation investigation on the default mode network involved in acupuncture: an fMRI study. Neurosci Lett. 2009;462(3):183–7.

Liu P, Zhou G, Zhang Y, et al. The hybrid GLM–ICA investigation on the neural mechanism of acupoint ST36: an fMRI study. Neurosci Lett. 2010;479(3):267–71.

Nomi JS, Farrant K, Damaraju E, et al. Dynamic functional network connectivity reveals unique and overlapping profiles of insula subdivisions. Hum Brain Mapp. 2016;37(5):1770–87.

Ptak R. The frontoparietal attention network of the human brain: action, saliency, and a priority map of the environment. Neuroscientist. 2012;18(5):502–15.

Qin W, Tian J, Bai L, et al. FMRI connectivity analysis of acupuncture effects on an amygdala-associated brain network. Mol Pain. 2008;13(4):55.

Seeley WW, Menon V, Schatzberg AF, et al. Dissociable intrinsic connectivity networks for salience processing and executive control. J Neurosci. 2007;27(9):2349–56.

Shen R, Taya F, Yu S, et al. Assessing small-worldness of dynamic functional brain connectivity during complex tasks. Conf Proc IEEE Eng Med Biol Soc. 2015;2015:2904–7.

Shi Y, Zhang S, Li Q, et al. A study of the brain functional network of Deqi via acupuncturing stimulation at BL40 by rs-fMRI. Complement Ther Med. 2016;25:71–7.

Thompson GJ, Merritt MD, Pan WJ, et al. Neural correlates of time-varying functional connectivity in the rat. NeuroImage. 2013;83:826–36.

Thompson GJ, Pan WJ, Magnuson ME, et al. Quasi-periodic patterns (QPP): large-scale dynamics in resting state fMRI that correlate with local infraslow electrical activity. NeuroImage. 2014;84:1018–31.

Viviani R. Emotion regulation, attention to emotion, and the ventral attentional network. Front Hum Neurosci. 2013;7:746.

Wang Z, Liang P, Zhao Z, et al. Acupuncture modulates resting state hippocampal functional connectivity in Alzheimer disease. PLoS One. 2014;9(3):e91160.

WHO. Acupuncture: review and analysis of reports on controlled clinical trials. Geneva: World Health Organization; 2002.

Wu MT, Sheen JM, Chuang KH, et al. Neuronal specificity of acupuncture response: a fMRI study with electroacupuncture. NeuroImage. 2002;16(4):1028–37.

Yoo J, Kim EY, Ahn YM, et al. Topological persistence vineyard for dynamic functional brain connectivity during resting and gaming stages. J Neurosci Methods. 2016;267:1–13.

Yoo SS, Teh EK, Blinder RA, et al. Modulation of cerebellar activities by acupuncture stimulation: evidence from fMRI study. NeuroImage. 2004;22(2):932–40.

Yu Q, Erhardt EB, Sui J, et al. Assessing dynamic brain graphs of time-varying connectivity in fMRI data: application to healthy controls and patients with schizophrenia. NeuroImage. 2015;107:345–55.

Zhang Y, Qin W, Liu P, et al. An fMRI study of acupuncture using independent component analysis. Neurosci Lett. 2009;449(1):6–9.

Zhong C, Bai L, Dai R, et al. Modulatory effects of acupuncture on resting-state networks: a functional MRI study combining independent component analysis and multivariate granger causality analysis. J Magn Reson Imaging. 2012;35(3):572–81.

Index

© Springer Nature Singapore Pte Ltd. 2018
J. Tian (ed.), *Multi-Modality Neuroimaging Study on Neurobiological Mechanisms of Acupuncture*, DOI 10.1007/978-981-10-4914-9

MIX
Papier aus verantwortungsvollen Quellen
Paper from responsible sources
FSC® C105338

If you have any concerns about our products,
you can contact us on
ProductSafety@springernature.com

In case Publisher is established outside the EU,
the EU authorized representative is:
Springer Nature Customer Service Center GmbH
Europaplatz 3, 69115 Heidelberg, Germany

Printed by Libri Plureos GmbH
in Hamburg, Germany